SpringerBriefs in Public Health

SpringerBriefs in Public Health present concise summaries of cutting-edge research and practical applications from across the entire field of public health, with contributions from medicine, bioethics, health economics, public policy, biostatistics, and sociology.

The focus of the series is to highlight current topics in public health of interest to a global audience, including health care policy; social determinants of health; health issues in developing countries; new research methods; chronic and infectious disease epidemics; and innovative health interventions.

Featuring compact volumes of 50 to 125 pages, the series covers a range of content from professional to academic. Possible volumes in the series may consist of timely reports of state-of-the art analytical techniques, reports from the field, snapshots of hot and/or emerging topics, elaborated theses, literature reviews, and in-depth case studies. Both solicited and unsolicited manuscripts are considered for publication in this series.

Briefs are published as part of Springer's eBook collection, with millions of users worldwide. In addition, Briefs are available for individual print and electronic purchase.

Briefs are characterized by fast, global electronic dissemination, standard publishing contracts, easy-to-use manuscript preparation and formatting guidelines, and expedited production schedules. We aim for publication 8–12 weeks after acceptance.

More information about this series at http://www.springer.com/series/10138

Muhammad Naveed Noor

Homeless Youth of Pakistan

Survival Sex and HIV Risk

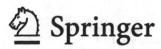

Muhammad Naveed Noor
Pathology & Laboratory Medicine
The Aga Khan University
Karachi, Pakistan

ISSN 2192-3698   ISSN 2192-3701   (electronic)
SpringerBriefs in Public Health
ISBN 978-3-030-79304-3   ISBN 978-3-030-79305-0   (eBook)
https://doi.org/10.1007/978-3-030-79305-0

This Springer imprint is published by the registered company Springer Nature Switzerland AG
The registered company address is: Gewerbestrasse 11, 6330 Cham, Switzerland

This book is dedicated to my parents for their immense love and encouragement to pursue my life goals.

Acknowledgements

This book emerged out of my PhD study, which I undertook from 2015 to 2019 at the University of New South Wales, Sydney, Australia. I acknowledge that I received enormous support from many people and institutions to conduct this study. First, I would like to express my deepest gratitude to my teachers – Associate Professor Joanne Bryant, Professor Martin Holt, and Professor John de Wit – for their excellent guidance, encouragement, and support (academic or otherwise), without which the timely completion of this study would not be possible. I also thank Dr Ayaz Qureshi from the University of Edinburgh, UK, for his brief but insightful comments on the analysis.

I acknowledge the valuable support and resources I received from the Centre for Social Research in Health, without which the research journey would have been much tougher. I am also indebted to the Higher Education Commission of Pakistan and the University of New South Wales for jointly providing me with funds to conduct this study.

I especially thank my wife Sunbal Fatima and my daughter Mairah Naveed Noor for their unfailing love and support. I also thank all my brothers and sisters, especially Dr Asia Noor for her kind wishes and support in pursuit of my dreams.

I am grateful to my study participants who provided rich insights into their life experiences, which rest at the heart of this book.

About the Book

While homeless young people (HYP) are typically perceived as *irresponsible* and *morally suspect* individuals who lack essential social skills to navigate their lives, this book offers an alternative and more positive perspective. It demonstrates that HYP improvise with resources available on the streets to improve their social and financial status, although they experience significant social structural constraints.

This ground-breaking book provides an analysis of social processes that contribute to young people's homelessness, their engagement in sex work, their establishment of intimate partnerships, and sexual practices, which may increase their risk of HIV and other sexually transmitted infections (STIs). The book demonstrates how the ongoing social and financial instability and insecurity neutralises HYP's knowledge of HIV/STIs, and how financial considerations, fear of violence by clients, and social obligations in intimate partnerships contribute to their sexual risk-taking. The author argues that the conventional approach of promoting health through raising awareness regarding HIV/STI prevention may continue to bring less than promising outcomes unless we focus on how structural and contextual conditions operate in the backdrop and produce conditions less conducive for young people.

Homeless Youth of Pakistan: Survival Sex and HIV Risk will attract undergraduate and postgraduate students as well as researchers interested in exploring issues such as youth homelessness, sexual risk-taking, and HIV/STIs.

Contents

About the Author

Muhammad Naveed Noor, MSc, MPhil, PhD is an assistant professor of health policy and system research at the Aga Khan University, Karachi, Pakistan. Dr Noor is trained in anthropology and social medicine. He received a PhD in social research in health from the University of New South Wales, Sydney, Australia. He contributed to various programmatic studies into maternal health, sexual and reproductive health, and women's dietary practices in the context of Pakistan. Dr Noor is currently part of an international team that investigates conflict of interest in medical profession and practice and how this contributes to overprescribing of antibiotics in Pakistan. Dr Noor can be reached at naveed.noor@aku.edu or m.noor@unswalumni.com.

About the Author

Chapter 1
Introduction

This book is about homeless young people (HYP) of Pakistan, who improvise with limited resources available on the street to obtain needed resources. While HYP are typically perceived as 'irresponsible' and 'morally suspect' individuals who lack essential social skills to navigate their lives, my analysis offers an alternative and more positive perspective. It suggests that HYP work in agential ways to address the problems that they face. One way by which HYP deal with these problems is to exchange sex for financial gains and social support, an activity that can reinforce their social marginalisation. In this introductory chapter – composed of two main parts – I set the scene for this book. In the first part, I provide an overview of the situation of HIV and youth homelessness in Pakistan. Here, I demonstrate the significance of conducting a social scientific study with HYP who often exchange sex for needed resources and how this places them at an increased risk of HIV and other sexually transmitted infections (STIs). In the second part, I provide a brief outline of the book structure.

Background

Due to a steady increase in the number of HIV cases over the last 30 years, HIV and other STIs have become key public health concerns in Pakistan. The first case of HIV in the country was reported in 1987, and since then, the epidemic has steadily expanded (Khan & Khan, 2010). During the initial years of HIV spread, HIV was generally considered a 'foreign disease', as most of the cases reported were either among foreigners living in Pakistan, or Pakistani migrants living and working overseas. In response to this, the National AIDS Control Program (NACP) was

© The Author(s), under exclusive license to Springer Nature Switzerland AG 2021
M. N. Noor, *Homeless Youth of Pakistan*, SpringerBriefs in Public Health,
https://doi.org/10.1007/978-3-030-79305-0_1

established in 1987 so that HIV diagnosis is improved and people living with HIV (PLWH) could receive adequate medical treatment. However, HIV was not a major concern in Pakistan until 2004 when it was found that 9.3% of people who injected drugs were seropositive in Sindh, the country's second-most populous province (Samo et al., 2013). Since then, national surveillance has found a consistent increase in the prevalence of HIV among other population groups, including transgender women, men who have sex with men, and female sex workers (Khan & Khan, 2010).

While HIV cases, during the last decade, have decreased by 0.7% per annum globally, the number of HIV cases in Pakistan has increased at an alarming rate of 9.1% per annum from 2005 to 2015 (UNAIDS, 2017). Additionally, the coverage of antiretroviral treatment (ART) – something that helps PLWH to live a healthier life – has remained, with recent estimates suggesting that only half of the registered PLWH regularly take ART (UNAIDS, 2018). As a consequence of low ART coverage, the death toll due to HIV/AIDS has increased from 250 in 2005 to 1480 in 2015 in Pakistan (Hussain et al., 2018). While the prevalence of HIV remains low in the general population in the country, the epidemic is well established and expanding among people who inject drugs (38.3%), transgender populations (7.5%), men who have sex with men (MSM) (3.4%), and female sex workers (2.1%) (NACP, 2017).

In developed country contexts, since the 1980s, homelessness has emerged as a critical social issue contributing to the increased prevalence of HIV (Torres et al., 1987). Studies have suggested that HYP are at far greater risk of HIV compared to their stably housed counterparts, largely due to a lack of access to HIV prevention and engaging in practices like injection drug use and risky sex (Boyer et al., 2017; Melander & Tyler, 2010). Given the circumstances surrounding discrimination and joblessness, HYP may engage in sex work – believed to be the most viable option for HYP to generate income, enough to meet their material needs, but it carries a high risk of HIV/STIs due to the chance of HYP inconsistently using condoms (Skyers et al., 2018).

Despite the relationship between HIV and social marginalisation, including homelessness, little is known about sexual practices among HYP in Pakistan – what they know about safe sex, how they make decisions about sex, and where they get help in their efforts to stay safe. To the best of my knowledge, this study is the first detailed social research to examine the social structural conditions that contribute to young people's homelessness, factors that shaped their sex work practices, their beliefs regarding sex and HIV/STIs, and reasons for using or not using condoms. Specifically, the study aimed to explore the social processes involved in shaping HYP's sexual practices that might increase their risk of HIV/STIs. The study was organised around the following research questions:

1. How do young people become homeless?
2. What strategies do HYP adopt to manage the difficult circumstances of their daily lives on the streets?
3. Why do HYP engage in sexual risk-taking, even when they know they are at risk of HIV/STIs?

Book Organisation

This book comprises nine chapters, including this introductory chapter.

Chapter 2, *Understanding Youth Homelessness*, describes past research into factors that contribute to youth homelessness and the strategies HYP employ to cope with adverse circumstances. This chapter is composed of two main parts. In the first part, I critically analyse past studies to identify what produces homelessness. The synthesis of multidisciplinary studies shows that homelessness can be better understood as a social situation produced through an interaction between micro-level factors, such as mental illness, drug/alcohol use, and physical/sexual violence, and macro-level factors, such as poverty, heteronormativity, and patriarchy. In the second part, I analyse research into the coping strategy of HYP. The analysis shows that HYP are agential, as they use various strategies (i.e. peer support, sex work, and the establishment of intimate partnerships) to improve their social and financial status within significant social structural constraints.

Chapter 3, *Understanding Sexual Behaviour*, attempts to analyse processes that shape sexual behaviour among young people. This chapter is composed of four major parts. In the first part, I examine beliefs that young people hold about sex and HIV/STIs and how they contradict biomedical knowledge. In the second part, I identify where beliefs about sex and HIV originate. In the third part, I review social psychology research to analyse the extent to which beliefs and/or biomedical knowledge about HIV/STIs shape sexual behaviour. In the fourth part, I review sociological studies to analyse how structural conditions can neutralise young people's beliefs and/or biomedical knowledge about sex and HIV/STIs and contribute to their sexual risk-taking.

Chapter 4, *The Theory of Capital and Social Practice*, describes the theoretical concepts used to explain the research findings. Pierre Bourdieu's theory of capital and social practice (1984 [1979]), comprised of three interrelated concepts of social fields, habitus, and capital, provides a relational view of social practice. Bourdieu (1998) proposes that society is a multidimensional space consisting of various subspaces called social fields such as family, religion, and education. Individuals enter these social fields with their unique habitus – competencies, worldviews, and perceived horizons of opportunity – and possess different forms of capital/resources. Every social field has an internal logic or set of rules called 'doxa' that gives individuals a sense of their own and others' positioning within a given social field. The habitus guides individuals in navigating social fields by shaping how they accumulate and deploy material, social, and cultural capital, a process which, on occasion, leads to social mobility or the acquisition of better social positions.

Chapter 5, *Methodological Approach to the Study*, is concerned with philosophical foundations that underpin the study and methods that I adopted to undertake it. The chapter is composed of two major parts. In the first part, I describe my ontological and epistemological stance. Based on the view that reality is socially constructed through the process of meaning-making, the study was underpinned by an idealist ontology and constructionist epistemology. In the second part, I give a brief overview of the study location and the methods adopted to conduct the study. In this part, I also discuss my fieldwork journey, data management and analysis, and how my position being an 'insider' and 'outsider' may have influenced the research process.

Chapter 6, *Capital Deficit and Youth Homelessness*, uses the concept of capital to analyse HYP's pathways to homelessness. This chapter is composed of four main parts. In the first part, I analyse how a lack of financial capital held by (rural) families and HYP's obligations to support poor parents shaped their decision to engage in paid work in an urban setting, and for this, they had to leave family homes. In the second part, I identify how families denied access to social capital to HYP with diverse sexual or gender identities; to secure which, they looked for other options of support outside family homes. In the third part, I analyse how, in some cases, domestic violence deteriorated family bond, and HYP thought to leave homes, even being cognisant of the risk of homelessness. In the fourth part, I analyse the role of illicit drug use in making family stop social capital supply to one homeless young man.

Chapter 7, *The Street Field: A Capital-Building Site*, describes various activities that HYP conducted to survive on the streets. This chapter has two main parts. In the first part, I analyse how HYP constructed a social space – which I call 'the street field' – and how this helped them to secure needed resources. In the second part, I describe how the street field was governed by certain rules and regulations and how they protected the existence of the street field and its members. The analysis here highlights HYP's agency – how they improvised with limited resources available on the streets to improve their social and financial status.

Chapter 8, *Sexual Risk-Taking: Competing Priorities of Capital-Building, Physical Safety, and Sexual Health*, considers how sex helped HYP to obtain social and financial resources but also carried the risks of HIV/STIs. This chapter has four main parts. In the first part, I highlight that HYP had concurrent sexual partnerships with clients and intimate partners. In the second part, I analysed the extent to which HYP were aware of sexual health risks and safety. Given the fact that HYP had reasonable knowledge about HIV/STIs, in the third part, I analysed factors that contributed to HYP's sexual risk-taking. In the fourth part, I show while HYP relied on some alternatives to reduce their risk of HIV/STIs, they were not biomedically effective. My analysis suggests that HYP's ongoing instability and insecurity inculcated into their habitus – the worldview that they had limited resources available on the streets and that losing intimate partners and clients would equate to losing social and financial capital. This context of competing priorities put HYP in a situation less conducive to condom use – something that increased HYP's risk of HIV/STIs.

Chapter 9, *Key Messages and Implications for Health Promotion*, describes the key contributions of the present study and its implications for policy, practice, and future research. This chapter is composed of four parts. In the first part, I describe key contributions of the study, especially how the theory of capital and social practice enabled the identification of social processes linked with homelessness and sexual risk-taking. In the second part, I reflect on some methodological aspects of the study. In the third part, in the light of the present study, I suggest some future areas of exploration in the country. In the fourth part, I demonstrate how 'five action areas' of the Ottawa Charter of Health Promotion can help reduce young people's risk of homelessness and HIV in Pakistan.

References

Bourdieu, P. (1984 [1979]). *Distinction: A social critique of the judgment of taste*. Harvard University Press.

Bourdieu, P. (1998). *On television* (P. P. Ferguson, Trans.). The New Press.

Boyer, C. B., Greenberg, L., Chutuape, K., Walker, B., Monte, D., Kirk, J., & Ellen, J. M. (2017). Exchange of sex for drugs or money in adolescents and young adults: An examination of sociodemographic factors, HIV-related risk, and community context. *Journal of Community Health, 42*, 90–100.

Hussain, A., Hussain, S., Ali, E., & Mehmood, A. (2018). HIV/AIDS – A growing epidemic in Pakistan. *Journal of Evolution of Medical and Dental Sciences, 7*(8), 1057–1062.

Khan, A. H., & Khan, A. (2010). The HIV epidemic in Pakistan. *Journal of the Pakistan Medical Association, 60*(4), 300–307.

Melander, L. A., & Tyler, K. A. (2010). The effect of early maltreatment, victimization, and partner violence on HIV risk behavior among homeless young adults. *Journal of Adolescent Health, 47*(6), 575–581.

NACP. (2017). *Integrated biological and behavioral surveillance in Pakistan 2016–17: 2nd generation HIV surveillance in Pakistan, round 5*. Retrieved from Islamabad.

Samo, R. N., Altaf, A., Agha, A., Pasha, O., Rozi, S., Memon, A., … Shah, A. (2013). High HIV incidence among persons who inject drugs in Pakistan: Greater risk with needle sharing and injecting frequently among the homeless. *PLoS One, 8*(12), e81715.

Skyers, N., Jarrett, S., McFarland, W., Cole, D., & Atkinson, U. (2018). HIV risk and gender in Jamaica's homeless population. *AIDS and Behavior, 22*, S65–S69.

Torres, R. A., Lefkowitz, P., Kales, C., & Brickner, P. W. (1987). Homelessness among hospitalized patients with the acquired immunodeficiency syndrome in New York City. *The Journal of the American Medical Association, 258*(6), 779–780.

UNAIDS. (2017). *Country factsheets, Pakistan*. Retrieved from www.unaids.org/en/regionscountries/countries/pakistan

UNAIDS. (2018). *Country progress report – Pakistan: Global AIDS Monitoring*. Retrieved from https://www.unaids.org/sites/default/files/country/documents/PAK_2018_countryreport.pdf

Chapter 2
Understanding Youth Homelessness

Homeless young people (HYP) often have lives characterised by inadequate social and financial resources, and this can contribute to their decisions to engage in survival sex. Therefore, to have a better understanding of HYP's sexual choices, decisions, and practices, it is important to explore factors that contribute to their homelessness in the first place. In this chapter, I review past research that attempts to understand young people's homelessness – how they become homeless and the resources they draw on to best cope with their homelessness. The chapter is composed of two major parts. In the first part, I review multidisciplinary studies to analyse how structural and interpersonal level forces interact to produce homelessness among HYP. In the second part, I review studies into HYP's survival strategies – how they make use of available resources to survive on the streets. The chapter closes with a discussion of how *the theory of capital and social practice* (Bourdieu, 1984 [1979], 1986) can be a valuable tool, not only to understand homelessness but also to highlight HYP's resourcefulness.

Youth Homelessness

The question of what produces homelessness in society does not have a straightforward answer. Indeed, explanations have been varied, with some researchers linking homelessness to broader social structures, some associating it with individuals' personal problems, and others establishing links across these antecedents. In earlier investigations, homelessness was portrayed in terms of individuals' disaffiliation from society, arising from personal problems such as mental health issues or illicit drug use; that is, they took a distinctly individualised approach to understand homelessness (Bahr, 1973). However, during the 1980s, the increased concentration of homeless people in major urban centres of the United States led social scientists to link the problem of homelessness with large-scale socioeconomic changes, such as

© The Author(s), under exclusive license to Springer Nature
Switzerland AG 2021
M. N. Noor, *Homeless Youth of Pakistan*, SpringerBriefs in Public Health,
https://doi.org/10.1007/978-3-030-79305-0_2

the deinstitutionalisation of health and social welfare systems, unemployment, unaffordable housing, and welfare budget cuts (Jencks, 1994). This historical shift was important in that researchers began to identify how macro-level forces operated to produce situations and contexts in which young people became homeless.

Nevertheless, in recent years, homelessness is seen to be a product of the relationship between individual personal pathologies and structural forces. Lee et al. (2010) suggest that macro-forces produce a population of people vulnerable to homelessness, where certain members of that at-risk population become homeless due to inadequate buffers. This scenario becomes evident when cross-disciplinary studies of homelessness are synthesised. While many studies draw linkages between childhood physical/sexual abuse and homelessness, the abuse itself is seen to be induced by how broader social structures operate in society. Researchers suggest that childhood physical/sexual abuse and negative family-related experiences, notably parental neglect, can negatively affect the family environment, resulting in youth leaving their homes (Tyler & Melander, 2012). Social psychology links the abuse and/or neglect with parents' mental illness or alcohol/drug use (Gelles, 1985; Murray, 1993; Zigler & Hall, 1989). These studies, however, do not adequately capture social structural forces that may lead to conditions where the abuse/neglect originates.

Sociological research suggests that parents' mental illness and/or their illicit drug/alcohol use may be a response to particular social structural problems. Parton (1985), for instance, in his book, *The Politics of Child Abuse*, describes how social class, gender, poverty, and other environmental conditions (such as the neighbourhood or community) influence the experience of child abuse in a family, which remains highly gendered, with rates of child abuse far higher for girls than for boys. Katz et al. (2007) argue that the relationship between poverty and child abuse is not straightforward, and it may be that financial hardship contributes to parent's mental stress, which may disrupt parenting practices.

Young people's mental illness has been highlighted as another important factor contributing to their homelessness. One view is that many people with mental illness choose to be alone as they experience difficulty in affiliating themselves with people in the family and workplace (Liegghio, 2017). Crane's (1998) study concerning the role of mental illness in homelessness in the UK has shown that young people's mental illness contributed to their disruption in familial ties, shaping their pathway to homelessness. However, Caton (1990) highlights the role of the deinstitutionalisation of mental health institutions in contributing to homelessness among a large number of people experiencing mental illness, notably in the United States, as the proponents of social treatment of mental illness believed that such people could receive better care in their families rather than in mental health institutions. Unfortunately, many of the people released from institutions found it very difficult to manage mental illness in the community, as did their families, contributing to a high rate of homelessness among former patients. In addition to this, social researchers like Joseph (2016) argue that the term 'mental illness' brings particular stigmatised, socially constructed meanings to people who are diagnosed and that these meanings impact their experiences, for instance, in navigating the healthcare system or society more generally.

Feminist research presents another perspective by offering gendered analyses of mental illness and homelessness and suggesting that a primary contributor to mental illness among women is the patriarchal structure of society (Balaa, 2014). For women, marital demands including the burden of household chores and childcare, in combination with the need for paid work, may negatively affect their mental health and well-being. Hamid et al. (2009), for instance, in their research on women in slum communities of Pakistan, found that some women reported experiencing verbal and/or physical abuse by husbands and/or in-laws if they did not provide expected levels of care to husbands and in-laws or conduct household chores. For Kazi et al. (2006), the abuse experienced by husbands and in-laws, together with the burden of household chores, may significantly contribute to depression among women, especially those who belong to lower social classes in Pakistan.

Similarly, heavy drug/alcohol use by young people is also identified as a significant contributor to their homelessness. Jencks (1994) viewed illicit drug/alcohol use as an individual pathology that hinders users from socioeconomic activities:

> Heavy [drug] use makes marginally employable adults even less employable, eats up money that would otherwise be available to pay rent, and makes their friends and relatives less willing to shelter them (Jencks, 1994, p. 44).

However, sociological research takes a broader approach by investigating why drug or alcohol use occurs in the first place. It attempts to draw linkages between broader social structures like poverty, gender, and young people's illicit drug or alcohol use (Spooner, 2009; Spooner & Hetherington, 2005). Researchers show that people who experience poverty and unemployment or have low levels of education are more likely to use illicit drugs and alcohol (Nagelhout et al., 2017). Quintero and Estrada (1998) link this issue with patriarchy, as they suggest that illicit drug use is a risk-taking practice and that risk-taking is associated with traditional forms of masculinity. Other studies suggest that illicit drug and alcohol use concentrates in social networks: young people whose family members or peers use illicit drugs or alcohol are more likely to do so (Aslund & Nilsson, 2013; Reynoso-Vallejo, 2011).

Homelessness as a growing issue for women has also been emphasised among homelessness researchers. One significant explanation of homelessness among women is marital or relationship breakdown (McDonald et al., 2007). While a marital breakdown is often portrayed as a micro-level issue because it involves conflict at the interpersonal level (i.e. the conflict between partners), social structural issues, notably poverty and patriarchy, can exacerbate it. According to Caton (1990), before becoming homeless, women often experience a disruption in family life, notably separation or divorce. Neale (1997) argues that in societies where women have insufficient financial resources, it may be more difficult for them to secure alternative accommodation arrangements after a relationship breakdown compared with men.

The relationship between economic factors and marriage breakdown is not straightforward because not all families with financial hardship experience breakdown. One view is that financial hardship can lead to tension between married couples, which can act as a basis for the breakdown of a marital relationship (Khan, 2001). Besides, according to Noble (1970), sociologists have sought to examine family breakdown concerning the sociocultural context in which it happens. Notably, patriarchy is given importance when it comes to feminist research, as Bettman (2009) suggests that domestic violence towards women largely stems from patriarchal social structures in society. Women may decide or feel that they have no choice but to leave home to escape abuse by their husband or partner (Baker et al., 2010).

In recent years, studies have highlighted how negative attitudes towards gender and sexual diversity can place people from sexual minorities at increased risk of homelessness. Researchers have suggested that people with gender and sexually diverse identities can face rejection when they disclose their sexual orientation or gender identity to their parents or others (Bird et al., 2017; Reck, 2009; Yadegarfard et al., 2014). This disclosure may affect the quality of young people's relationships with their parents and manifest in decreased care, concern, and warmth. The main reason behind the familial rejection of gender and sexually diverse people has been attributed to homophobia, biphobia, and transphobia reinforced by heteronormativity – a social structure that positions heterosexuality as the only natural, unquestioned, and normal way of expressing as well as practising sexuality and is maintained by social institutions like marriage, religion, and the law (Bird et al., 2017). The power associated with heteronormativity can lead to the marginalisation of those who do not conform to such norms.

In short, although micro-level issues such as mental illness, childhood physical/sexual abuse, domestic violence against women, and rejection of diverse gender and sexual identities contribute to young people's homelessness, these issues are linked with macro-structures like poverty, patriarchy, and heteronormativity. Therefore, homelessness can perhaps be best understood through a relational lens: an entanglement of both macro-structural and micro-individual/interpersonal factors and the approach that will be taken in this study.

Survival Strategies

Since HYP may possess limited social and financial resources and are often aware that society perceives them as 'irresponsible and dangerous', an important way for them to obtain social support is to remain connected to peers who understand or share their circumstances and are not negatively judgmental of their situation (Lee et al., 2010, p. 508). In his research from Australia, Barker (2012, 2013) used the concept of social capital and suggested that because HYP's lives can be characterised by the lack of social capital, they attempt to accumulate and preserve their social capital by establishing peer networks. He further describes how peers provided HYP with social, emotional, and, sometimes, financial support, absent from their family lives.

Lee et al. (2010) suggest that together, disruption in family ties, social stigma associated with homelessness, and, sometimes, verbal/physical abuse by the general public contribute to HYP's emotional distress. Here, peer networks can play an important role to reduce their emotional distress, notably by providing care and help to secure shelter, food, and paid work. For example, Watson (2011), in her research from Australia, demonstrates how intimate partners provided homeless young women with a range of capital and resources essential to survive in homelessness:

> For young women experiencing homelessness, an intimate relationship can offer economic capital in the form of material support, cultural capital through the affirmation of femininity, and social capital through possible access to increased networks and resources. (p. 643)

Researchers like Beazley (2003) and Davies (2008) suggest that on the streets young people may develop a distinct sub-culture operating parallel to the predominating culture of a given society. This sub-culture may promote things like illicit drug/alcohol use and violence against the general public as a way to respond to the social stigma associated with homelessness and to foster their identity. In social psychology research, these practices are understood as emotion-focused coping strategies, which are used to reduce emotional distress associated with the condition of homelessness (Dashora et al., 2016; Opalach et al., 2016). However, social research suggests that practices like the use of illicit drug/alcohol can be understood as a form of capital – the cultural capital, which HYP often use to test their physical strength, to create a sense of belonging to a sub-culture, to stop hunger pains, to gain pleasure, and to cope with emotional distress (Beazley, 2003; Davies, 2008).

Other studies have investigated the reasons behind HYP's use of violence. In these studies, a predominant view is that since HYP know that they are perceived to be morally suspect and dangerous individuals, there may be increased chances of experiencing violence by the general public (Alverdinia & Pridemore, 2012; Sandberg, 2008; Tyler & Melander, 2012). Therefore, HYP use aggression and violence against the general public to deter potential incidents of abuse from them. Indeed, the use of violence against the general public can permit HYP to see themselves as having a sense of control, power, and dignity (Lee et al., 2011). However, Barker (2013) uses the concept of 'negative cultural capital' (p. 358) to suggest that HYP's use of aggression and violence can be understood in terms of their cultural competence, which they use to attain a social status so that they feel less marginalised. This cultural capital, from the perspective of the general public, may be perceived negatively – something that reinforces their social marginalisation.

HYP may also develop specific symbolic identities as a way to challenge the conventional norms of society. Beazley (2003) uses the term 'specialised semiotic' to refer to how the street sub-culture in Indonesia requires that its members should look different to the general public. She found that HYP underwent body modifications, such as tattooing and piercing, to feel a sense of belonging with each other and to feel part of a sub-culture in defiance of broader Indonesian society. In the same vein, Davies (2008), in his research from Kenya, found how HYP use specific slangs (which are usually not understandable by the general public), body gestures like clapping, finger clicking, and slapping the knees or the ground, all of which convey particular meanings, to have a sense of shared identity. Davies (2008) also describes that his research participants wore specific outfits – long coats with patchwork, which helped them to conceal things like money, food, dice, cards, and drugs.

Since HYP often have trouble in finding jobs in the formal market, partly due to social stigma attached to homelessness, they are seen to be engaged with what Snow and Anderson (1993, p. 145) refer to as 'shadow work': theft, drug sales, and survival sex. Researchers suggest that often among HYP, engagement in sex work is given primacy, as it is considered the most viable way to generate income, enough to meet their material needs (Asante et al., 2014; Mayock et al., 2013). However, engagement in sex work is of course associated with negative physical and social consequences – stigmatisation, social exclusion, and unprotected sex (Barman-Adhikari et al., 2017; Purser et al., 2017).

Overall, studies reviewed in this section suggest that HYP can devise creative ways to deal with significant social structural constraints they face in their everyday lives. Indeed, studies show that they improvise with limited resources available on the streets to secure the resources they need to survive in homelessness. While coping strategies outlined above can be strategic ways for HYP to attain things like physical protection, having a sense of shared identity, self-worth, and money, these practices are often stigmatising. Indeed, the review shows that these practices, from the perspective of the general public, are perceived to be anti-social – something that reinforces HYP's social marginalisation.

Conclusion

In this chapter, I have reviewed past research into young people's pathways to homelessness and their survival strategies. The review suggests that homelessness may be better understood in terms of a product of interaction between micro- and macro-level social forces. It shows that while individuals' personal problems like mental illness and illicit drug/alcohol use, and sometimes social interaction, at the interpersonal level, do contribute to young people's homelessness, these issues work together with social structural issues like poverty, gender, heteronormativity, and patriarchy. Studies reviewed in the second section demonstrate the agential ways in which HYP deal with significant social structural constraints they face in their everyday lives. Specifically, studies show that HYP establish peer networks, use drugs, unleash violence against the general public, and practise sex work to secure physical protection and to have a sense of identity and other material resources essential to survive homelessness. However, these practices are often counter-productive because of how they are perceived by the general public, and this can reinforce HYP's social marginalisation.

References

Alverdinia, A., & Pridemore, W. A. (2012). Individual-level factors contributing to homelessness among adult males in Iran. *Sociological Spectrum, 32*(3), 209–225.

Asante, K. O., Meyer-Weitz, A., & Petersen, I. (2014). Substance use and risky sexual behaviours among street connected children and youth in Accra, Ghana. *Substance Abuse Treatment, Prevention & Policy, 9*, 45.

Aslund, C., & Nilsson, K. W. (2013). Social capital in relation to alcohol consumption, smoking, and illicit drug use among adolescents: A cross-sectional study in Sweden. *International Journal for Equity in Health, 12*, 33.

Bahr, H. M. (1973). *Skid row: An introduction to disaffiliation*. Oxford University Press.

Baker, C. K., Billhardt, K. A., Warren, J., Rollins, C., & Glass, N. E. (2010). Domestic violence, housing instability, and homelessness: A review of housing policies and program. *Aggression and Violent Behaviour, 15*, 430–439.

Balaa, L. (2014). Why insanity is not subversive in Hanan Al-Shaykh's short story 'season of madness'. *Australian Feminist Studies, 29*(82), 480–499.

Barker, J. D. (2012). Social capital, homeless young people and the family. *Journal of Youth Studies, 15*(6), 730–743.

Barker, J. D. (2013). Negative cultural capital and homeless young people. *Journal of Youth Studies, 16*(3), 358–374.

Barman-Adhikari, A., Hasu, H. T., Begun, S., Portillo, A. P., & Rice, E. (2017). Condomless sex among homeless youth: The role of multidimensional social norms and gender. *AIDS Behavior, 21*, 688–702.

Beazley, H. (2003). Voices from the margins: Street children's subcultures in Indonesia. *Children's Geographies, 1*(2), 181–200.

Bettman, C. (2009). Patriarchy: The predominant discourse and fount of domestic violence. *The Australian and New Zealand Journal of Family Therapy, 30*(1), 15–18.

Bird, J. P., Sala, M. C., Hidalgo, M. A., Kuhns, L. M., & Garofalo, R. (2017). "I Had to Go to the Streets to Get Love": Pathways from parental rejection to HIV risk among young gay and bisexual men. *Journal of Homosexuality, 64*(3), 321–342.

Bourdieu, P. (1984 [1979]). *Distinction: A social critique of the judgment of taste*. Harvard University Press.

Bourdieu, P. (1986). The forms of capital. In J. G. Richardson (Ed.), *Handbook of theory and research for the sociology* (pp. 241–258). Greenwood.

Caton, C. L. (1990). *Homeless in America*. Oxford University Press.

Crane, M. (1998). The associations between mental illness and homelessness people: An exploratory study. *Aging & Mental Health, 2*(3), 171–180.

Dashora, P., Erdem, G., & Slesnick, N. (2016). Better to bend than to break: Coping strategies utilized by substance-abusing homeless youth. *Journal of Health Psychology, 16*(1), 158–168.

Davies, M. (2008). Childish Culture? Shared understandings, agency and intervention: An anthropological study of street children in Northwest Kenya. *Childhood. SAGE Publications, 15*(3), 309–330.

Gelles, R. J. (1985). Family violence. *Annual Review of Sociology, 11*, 347–367.

Hamid, S., Johansson, E., & Rubenson, B. (2009). "Who am I? Where am I?" Experiences of married young women in a slum in Islamabad, Pakistan. *BMC Public Health, 9*(1), 265.

Jencks, C. (1994). *The homeless*. Harvard University Press.

Joseph, M. J. (2016). Is mental illness socially constructed? *Journal of Applied Psychology and Social Science, 2*(1), 1–11.

Katz, I., Corlyon, J., Placa, V. L., & Hunter, S. (2007). *The relationship between parenting and poverty*. Retrieved from https://www.jrf.org.uk/sites/default/files/jrf/migrated/files/parenting-poverty.pdf

Kazi, A., Fatmi, Z., Hatcher, J., Kadir, M. M., Niaz, U., & Wasserman, G. A. (2006). Social environment and depression among pregnant women in urban areas of Pakistan: Importance of social relations. *Social Science & Medicine, 63*(6), 1466–1476.

Khan, S. (2001). *The nature and causes of marital breakdown amongst a selected group of South African Indian Muslims in the Durban Metropolitan area and its consequences for family life*. University of Durban-Westville.

Lee, B. A., Tyler, K. A., & Wright, J. D. (2010). The new homelessness revisited. *Annual Review of Sociology, 36*, 501–521.

Lee, S.-J., Liang, L.-J., Rotheram-Borus, M. J., & Milburn, N. G. (2011). Resiliency and survival skills among newly homeless adolescents: Implications for future interventions. *Vulnerable Children and Youth Studies, 6*(4), 301–308.

Liegghio, M. (2017). 'Not a good person': Family stigma of mental illness from the perspectives of young siblings. *Child and Family Social Work, 22*(3), 1237–1245.

Mayock, P., Corr, L. M., & O'Sullivan, E. (2013). Moving on, not out: When young people remain homeless. *Journal of Youth Studies, 16*(4), 441–459.

McDonald, L., Dergal, J., & Cleghorn, L. (2007). Living on the margins. *Journal of Gerontological Social Work, 49*(1–2), 19–46.

Murray, J. B. (1993). Relationship of childhood sexual abuse to borderline personality disorder, posttraumatic stress disorder, and multiple personality disorder. *The Journal of Psychology, 127*(6), 657–676.

Nagelhout, G. E., Hummel, K., De Goeij, M. C., De Vries, H., Kaner, E., & Lemmens, P. (2017). How economic recessions and unemployment affect illegal drug use: A systematic realist literature review. *International Journal of Drug Policy, 44*, 69–83.

Neale, J. (1997). Theorising homelessness, contemporary sociological, and feminist perspective. In R. Burrows, N. Pleace, & D. Quilgars (Eds.), *Homelessness and social policy*. Routledge.

Noble, T. (1970). Family breakdown and social networks. *The British Journal of Sociology, 21*(2), 135–150.

Opalach, C., Romaszko, J., Jaracz, M., Kuchta, R., Borkowska, A., & Bucinski, A. (2016). Coping styles and alcohol dependence among homeless people. *PLoS One, 11*(9), e0162381.

Parton, N. (1985). *The politics of child abuse*. Macmillan.

Purser, G. L., Mowbray, O. P., & O'Shields, J. (2017). The relationship between length and number of homeless episodes and engagement in survival sex. *Journal of Social Service Research, 43*(2), 262–269.

Quintero, G. A., & Estrada, A. L. (1998). Cultural models of masculinity and drug use: "machismo," heroin, and street survival on the U.S.-Mexico border. *Contemporary Drug Problems, 25*(1), 147–168.

Reck, J. (2009). Homeless gay and transgender youth of color in San Francisco: "No one likes street kids"—Even in the Castro. *Journal of LGBT Youth, 6*(2–3), 223–242.

Reynoso-Vallejo, H. (2011). Social capital influence in illicit drug use among racial/ethnic groups in the United States. *Journal of Ethnicity in Substance Abuse, 10*(2), 91–111.

Sandberg, S. (2008). Street capital, ethnicity and violence on the streets of Oslo. *Theoretical Criminology, 12*(2), 153–171.

Snow, D. A., & Anderson, L. (1993). *Down on their luck: A study of homeless street people*. University of California Press.

Spooner, C. (2009). Social determinants of drug use – Barriers to translating research into policy. *Health Promotion Journal of Australia, 20*(3), 180–185.

Spooner, C., & Hetherington, C. (2005). *Social determinants of drug use*. Retrieved from Sydney.

Tyler, A. K., & Melander, A. L. (2012). Poor parenting and antisocial behaviour among homeless young adults: Links to dating violence perpetration and victimization. *Journal of Interpersonal Violence, 27*(7), 1357–1373.

Watson, J. (2011). Understanding survival sex: Young women, homelessness and intimate relationships. *Journal of Youth Studies, 14*(6), 639–655.

Yadegarfard, M., Meinhold-Bergmann, M. E., & Ho, R. (2014). Family rejection, social isolation, and loneliness as predictors of negative health outcomes (depression, suicidal ideation, and sexual risk behavior) among Thai male-to-female transgender adolescents. *Journal of LGBT Youth, 11*(4), 347–363.

Zigler, E., & Hall, N. W. (1989). Physical child abuse in America: Past, present and future. In D. Cicchetti & V. Carlson (Eds.), *Child maltreatment: Theory and research on the causes and consequences of child abuse and neglect* (pp. 38–75). Cambridge University Press.

Chapter 3
Understanding Sexual Behaviour

Homeless young people (HYP) are often seen to be engaging in sexual risk-taking due to their limited knowledge about sexual health risks and safety. However, recent social research suggests that individuals' knowledge of sexual health risks and safety may not always help them to avoid sexual health risks. Indeed, various social structural and contextual factors may operate to shape their sexual choices, decisions, and practices. In this chapter, I review studies about young people's beliefs about sex and HIV and other sexually transmitted infection (STIs), the relationship between those beliefs and sexual behaviour as well as social structural conditions and sexual behaviour.

This chapter is composed of four main sections. In the first section, I review studies regarding young people's beliefs about transmission, infectiousness, and the prevention of HIV/STIs. The review in this section indicates that young people often hold beliefs that do not align with biomedical knowledge regarding HIV/STIs. In the second section, I review studies that investigate where these beliefs about sex and HIV/STIs originate. This review shows how a combination of structural and interpersonal level forces produce beliefs that contradict biomedical knowledge of sexual health risks and safety. In the third section, I review studies from social psychology that explore the relationship between beliefs about sex and HIV/STIs and sexual behaviour. This review indicates that explanations of whether beliefs impact sexual behaviour are inconsistent, with some of them providing hints of how social structural forces can constrain individuals' sexual behaviour. Therefore, in the fourth section, I review research that explores the relationships between structural conditions and sexual behaviour. This review in this section suggests that various social structures, which are intricately linked with the production of HIV/STIs beliefs, can also constrain sexual behaviour so that young people use condoms inconsistently, despite being aware of the risk of HIV/STIs. The chapter closes with the discussion of how the theory of capital and social practice (Bourdieu, 1984 [1979], 1986) is well suited to explain why knowledge regarding HIV/STIs may not always help young people to practise safer sex. Specifically, the theory can help to

M. N. Noor, *Homeless Youth of Pakistan*, SpringerBriefs in Public Health, https://doi.org/10.1007/978-3-030-79305-0_3

understand how social, cultural, and financial resources may produce contexts where young people may engage in sexual risk-taking, even while being cognisant of the risk of HIV/STIs.

Beliefs About HIV/STIs

In the 1980s, HIV was identified as the cause of AIDS and became a global epidemic that contributed to morbidity and mortality across the world due to the absence of widespread access to prevention methods and a lack of effective treatments (Gross & Tyring, 2011). A steady increase in the number of HIV cases each year in the following decades resulted in HIV/STIs becoming key public health concerns globally. However, since the late 1990s, HIV can be successfully treated by antiretroviral drugs, although the infection cannot be eliminated (Ford et al., 2018).

Advances in biomedical research have increased our understanding of the transmission, prevention, and treatment of HIV/STIs (Cowan & Bell, 2011). For instance, while HIV remains a major global cause of mortality, the introduction of combination antiretroviral treatment (ART) has led to a dramatic decrease in HIV-related deaths all over the world, since ART can suppress HIV replication, leading to an undetectable viral load (Williams et al., 2011). Furthermore, in the recent era, pre-exposure prophylaxis (PrEP), the regular use of antiretroviral drugs by HIV-negative people to prevent HIV acquisition, has been found to be highly effective in preventing HIV infection (Fonner et al., 2016).

Additionally, health promotion campaigns in many countries have attempted to educate people about health risks and promote condom use in particular to prevent the sexual transmission of HIV/STIs (Delobelle et al., 2010). Despite these efforts, the rates of HIV/STIs have been increasing globally. According to recent global estimates, the number of people living with HIV (PLWH) has increased from 27.4 million in 2000 to almost 37.0 million in 2017, although this is not a failure, as the use of ART in the recent era is keeping most of the PLWH alive (UNAIDS, 2018). Similarly, while the National AIDS Control Program of Pakistan (NACP) has been educating the general public about HIV infection, HIV incidence is increasing, particularly among key populations that include people who inject drugs, transgender women, men who have sex with men, and sex workers (NACP, 2014).

Social researchers like Warwick et al. (1988), nearly three decades ago, turned their attention to exploring individuals' 'lay' beliefs regarding HIV/AIDS. Their research aimed to provide recommendations for designing effective HIV prevention interventions, notably in African countries, where HIV affected thousands of people in that era. Since then, studies have been highlighting beliefs that people hold regarding the causes, infectiousness, transmission, prevention, and treatment of HIV/STIs. For instance, in exploring beliefs about HIV among young Muslim women living in Australia, Meldrum et al. (2016) found that a few women considered HIV as a form of cancer rather than a virus that can be transmitted sexually

(p. 131). Nicoll et al. (1993) found that people including some healthcare workers in East Africa believed that HIV had occurred accidentally – HIV, originally, was an organism that caused leprosy. People affected by leprosy were killed during the war between Uganda and Tanzania and fell into Lake Victoria. Since those people were eaten by fish and the leprosy organism was converted into HIV, people who ate those fish contracted HIV. Other researchers have reported how young people from African countries, as well as African Americans, hold conspiracy beliefs about the origin of HIV. In the context of Uganda, Mutonyi et al. (2010) found that young people believed that HIV was invented in a laboratory in the United States and used as a 'weapon of mass destruction' (p. 582) against African people.

Young people's beliefs about the causes of HIV have also been explored. For example, some studies from African countries show that, in addition to misfortune, people believe that witchcraft, sorcery, and curses from ancestral spirits cause HIV infection (Longfield et al., 2003; Mshana et al., 2006; Nuwaha et al., 2001). In the context of Zambia, researchers found that one-fifth of the sampled young people associated HIV/AIDS with witchcraft (Menon et al., 2015).

Young people are seen to hold different beliefs about sexual behaviours that can cause HIV infection. When HIV is viewed through a conservative or traditional moral lens, people believe that HIV is a divine punishment for those involved in sexual practices that are often forbidden or discouraged (like having sex outside marriage or sex between men) from the perspective of religion (Andrinopoulos et al., 2011). Another consistent finding across these studies is that young people may believe that HIV can spread through casual contacts, such as touching PLWH. For instance, in a study from Botswana, researchers found that young people believed that kissing, hugging, shaking hands, and sharing utensils with HIV-positive people could transmit HIV (Nleya & Segale, 2015).

Nleya and Segale (2015) suggest that although young people may know that HIV can be transmitted through condomless sex with an infected partner, they may also hold inaccurate beliefs about alternative modes of transmission. Scholars, notably from developing country contexts, suggest a persistent belief that mosquito bites can transmit HIV (Kang et al., 2017). A study in East Africa by Nicoll et al. (1993) revealed that this belief continued to persist among some health workers despite national health promotion campaigns.

Some researchers like Dunn et al. (2017) found that female sex workers believed that the use of antibiotics and vaginal douching could prevent their risk of HIV/STIs while having condomless sex with clients. Similarly, Nleya and Segale (2015) found that teachers and students in Botswana believed that HIV could be prevented by drinking a lot of water after having sex.

While there is a relative dearth of research into beliefs about HIV/STIs in Pakistan, a few studies have shown how similar to other parts of the world, young people in Pakistan hold beliefs that contradict accepted scientific knowledge of HIV/STIs. Raza et al. (1998) conducted survey research with 1088 young people in Pakistan and found that, like other developing countries, the study participants believed that mosquito bites and touching a PLWH could transmit HIV. Also, Abrar and Ghouri (2010) found that young people in Pakistan linked HIV to malnutrition and also believed that using the same toilet as a PLWH could transmit HIV. Similarly, Raheel et al. (2007) found that university students in Pakistan believed that HIV infection was highly infectious, as it was thought to spread through the air, through sharing toilets, or through sharing utensils with PLWH.

Studies reviewed in this section suggest that despite health promotion efforts, which may be inadequate, particularly in developing countries, young people across the world may hold beliefs that do not necessarily align with biomedical knowledge of HIV/STIs. To provide recommendations for culturally appropriate intervention, social researchers like Warwick et al. (1988) have explored where these beliefs orig- inate, a detailed description of which is provided in the next section.

The Origins of Beliefs About HIV/STIs

Beliefs about HIV/STIs are thought to be better understood in terms of local cultural knowledge. Indeed, the cultural background is seen to be playing a critical role in how sex and sexual health risks may be perceived in a given community (Meldrum et al., 2016). Recent social research suggests that this local cultural knowledge, notably about sex and HIV, can be understood as a product of entanglement between micro- and macro-level social forces, what they call 'the middle ground of social practice' (Kippax et al., 2013, p. 1367). These researchers argue that individuals, in a given community, generally act as the members of collectives, implying that social interaction primarily shapes how to perceive things and act in society. However, these perceptions and practices typically align with and reinforce community norms promoted by predominant social structures. For instance, individuals' relationships with people they are close to and whom they trust, particularly family members and friends, can play a critical role in shaping their understanding of HIV/STIs (Byron, 2017). Based on information derived from social networks, young people see HIV infection as a result of morality rather than inconsistent condom use (Mmari et al., 2016).

Sociological research demonstrates how social structures like conservative reli- gion and heteronormativity create links between HIV/STIs and morality. For instance, some researchers suggest religious faith can influence the belief that HIV is divine punishment against those who transgress socioreligious norms relating to sex (Bello, 2011; Garofalo et al., 2015). Religion can unite people into a moral com- munity that holds certain beliefs and obligations. In most of the world's major reli- gions, including Islam, Christianity, and Hinduism, practices like sex outside of marriage and homosexuality are prohibited and held up as examples of moral weak- ness or degeneracy (Adamczyk & Hayes, 2012). Studies have found that Muslims and Hindus tend to have more conservative attitudes towards such sexual practices than Christians and Jews (Addai, 2000; Agha, 2009; Finke & Adamczyk, 2008).

The response of religious denominations to HIV/AIDS has been an important characteristic of the global response to the epidemic. According to Adamczyk and

Hayes (2012), religion influences people's attitudes towards sexuality and these attitudes are passed on and rehearsed in interpersonal relationships. Since most of the world's major religions are critical of practices like sex outside marriage and homosexual sex, religious leaders have sometimes interpreted HIV/AIDS in terms of divine punishment for moral weakness or failure to observe religious doctrine and have propagated this belief to their followers (Maulana et al., 2009). Therefore, the stigma associated with HIV/AIDS is often seen to be manifested in 'verbal abuse, gossip, and distancing from people living with HIV/AIDS' (Liamputtong, 2013, p. 3).

Because Pakistan is an Islamic country, society, culture, and law promote Islamic teachings in all values and codes that guide and influence individuals' everyday lives (Qadir et al., 2005). Therefore, following Islamic principles, practices like sex outside marriage and same-sex sex are prohibited and people who transgress these socioreligious norms of sexuality can experience stigmatisation, discrimination, and expulsion from families and even can be prosecuted under the law (Rajabali et al., 2008). Also, similar to Catholic and Protestant leaders in other parts of the world, religious leaders in Pakistan argue against sex education and the promotion of condom use, as they believe that promoting these will undermine religious morality and lead to societal degradation (Oluduro, 2010, p. 215). In their research with young people in Pakistan, Abrar and Ghouri (2010) found that based on information derived from religious leaders, most participants linked HIV with 'sexual deviance/ homosexuality' (p. 272).

Religion is also considered an important social structure in the enforcement of heteronormativity, which reinforces a belief that practising homosexuality is wrong and can cause HIV (Henshaw, 2014). The concept of heteronormativity is used to highlight the social construction of human sexuality and refers to ways in which heterosexuality is constructed and performed as the natural and normal way of expressing and practising sexuality, which is maintained by social institutions such as marriage, the law, and family (Herz & Johansson, 2015). Within heteronormative societies and structures, other forms of sexuality (such as homosexuality) are positioned as deviant and dangerous to population well-being, justifying regulation, monitoring, and intervention (Foucault, 1990).

Studies reviewed in this section highlight how a combination of micro- and macro-level forces produce beliefs about HIV/STIs. Specifically, it shows that social structures like religion and heteronormativity link sex outside marriage and sex between men with morality, something which is reinforced in everyday micro-level social interactions. My analysis reveals that young people hold beliefs that may or may not align with biomedical knowledge about HIV/STIs and how the beliefs may be shaped by health promotion and dominant structures of religion and heteronormativity. This exposition raises an important question as to what extent young people's understanding of HIV/STIs can shape their sexual practices, which the next section attempts to address.

The Extent to Which Beliefs Shape Sexual Behaviour

In explaining individuals' sexual behaviours and designing potentially effective interventions, researchers have mainly relied on social psychological theories, in particular the health belief model (HBM), social cognitive theory (SCT), the theory of reasoned action (TRA) and its successor, the theory of planned behaviour (TPB), and the prototype willingness model (PWM) (Conner & Norman, 2015). The key constructs used in social psychological theories include perceived susceptibility (from HBM), intention to perform a specific behaviour that depends on individuals' attitudes and subjective norms (from TRA and TPB), perceived outcome (from HBM and SCT), self-efficacy or behavioural control beliefs (from TPB and SCT), and structural/environmental constraints (from SCT).

Given the overlap and similarity between various variables in social psychological theories, researchers have attempted to develop an integrated behavioural model (IBM) (Conner & Norman, 2015). The IBM includes eight key constructs. It posits that for individuals to perform a specific behaviour, they must have a strong intention, knowledge, and skills sufficient to perform that behaviour, and there must be an absence of environmental constraints that may prevent that behaviour. Furthermore, for individuals to have a strong behavioural intention, they must perceive the benefits of performing the intended behaviour, have a high level of self-efficacy, have a belief that the intended behaviour complies with their self-image, have positive emotions about the intended behaviour, and perceive increased social pressure to perform the intended behaviour (Conner & Norman, 2015).

Drawing on the aforementioned key theories and their constructs, researchers have attempted to provide recommendations for potentially effective interventions to promote behaviours inclined towards better health outcomes. However, there has been little consensus on what theories and constructs are well suited to explain individuals' health behaviours. For instance, drawing on the TPB, Villarruel et al. (2004) analysed the likelihood of Spanish young people's intention to have sexual intercourse. In this study, subjective norms were associated with young people's intentions to have sex. Young people who believed their parents were not supportive of their engagement in sex were more likely to abstain from sex. Gillmore et al. (2002), in their study from the United States, found young people's attitudes towards sexual risks to be associated with their sexual behaviour rather than subjective norms. Young people who believed that sexual intercourse could lead to negative outcomes, such as unwanted pregnancy or STIs, were more likely to use condoms. Widman et al. (2013), however, in their study from the United States, found that self-efficacy was associated with condom use among young PLWH. Importantly, studies employing IBM have shown that attitudes, subjective norms, behavioural control, and the absence of environmental constraints all may be associated with condom use, depending on the context (Kasprzyk et al., 1998; Von Haeften & Kensk, 2001).

Researchers have also compared social psychological theories to analyse which theory/model is better suited to explain individuals' sexual behaviour. For instance, Vanlandingham et al. (1995) compared the TRA and the HBM to determine the likelihood of condom use among men in Northern Thailand. They found that TRA explained Thai men's sexual behaviour better than the HBM. In contrast, Montanaro and Bryan (2014) compared the TPB and the HBM to analyse the likelihood of condom use among university students in the United States. This study found that the TPB was better suited to explain the likelihood of students' condom use than HBM.

While Taylor et al. (2006) have suggested that the TRA and the TPB have the same predictive power, Tyson et al. (2014) have found that the TPB is more useful to explain people's condom use and, therefore, is an important tool to develop potentially useful interventions. Sheeran and Taylor (1999) emphasised the construct of perceived behavioural control from the TPB. They suggested that perceived behavioural control was associated with people's behavioural intentions and explained more variance in condom use as compared to attitudes and subjective norms. On the other hand, Gebhardt et al. (2009), in their 1-year follow-up study with female undergraduate students from the Netherlands, suggested that the PWM explained more variance in condom use than the TPB. Wulfert and Wan (1995) used the HBM, TRA, and SCT to explain the likelihood of condom use among older adults and college students in the United States and found SCT to be more useful, as the theory explained 70% variance in intentions to use condoms among older adults. Wulfert and Wan (1995) longitudinally tested the SCT with sexually active students, explaining a 50% variance in condom use. While the use of the aforementioned models provides insights into cognitive processes, it does not help to analyse structural and contextual factors that may play a critical role in shaping individuals' sexual behaviour.

Thus, studies reviewed in this section illustrate the range of cognitive processes and social norms that can shape individuals' sexual choices, decisions, and practices. Nevertheless, the analysis suggests that research findings from social psychological studies are inconsistent rather than revealing universal mechanisms underpinning health behaviours. Also, it does not adequately explain how various contextual and structural factors like the role of sociosexual norms, heteronormativity, and patriarchy can constrain individuals' sexual behaviour. Therefore, the next section reviews sociological research to identify the role of contextual and structural factors like poverty, social obligations, religion, heteronormativity, and patriarchy on young people's sexual behaviour.

Sexual Behaviour and Structural Conditions

Sociological perspectives suggest that beliefs about sex and sexual health risks are not always so directly predictive of practices and other factors that may contribute to individuals' engagement in sexual behaviour, and particularly sex that may be risky for HIV/STIs. Researchers have shown that despite being cognisant of sexual health risks, young people may engage in concurrent sexual partnerships (Garofalo et al., 2015). One perspective is that in male-dominant societies, men will generally practise sex outside marriage, as practices like sexual abstinence and monogamy are often considered emasculating (Ussher et al., 2012). Also, there is evidence of a massive double standard when it comes to women's engagement in premarital sex in conservative societies. Notably, in Islamic societies, women are expected to preserve their virginity until they get married, and going against this norm may lead women to experience stigmatisation. Hamid et al. (2010) suggest that in Pakistan, young women are generally discouraged to receive education regarding sexuality, as 'sexual innocence' (p. 1) of women is considered a sign of purity – something that largely stems from predominant sociocultural and religious discourses in the country. Therefore, women belonging to conservative societal origins and living in developed world settings are not encouraged to receive sex education and engage in premarital sex. For example, in their study with young Muslim women living in Australia, Meldrum et al. (2014) found that women believed that irrespective of physical desire to have sex, they did not do so because women's engagement in premarital sex could affect their reputation as 'pure' women (p. 175). Here, many scholars emphasise the dominant nature of the patriarchal social structure that often validates men's sexual promiscuousness while suppressing women's sexual autonomy (MacPhail & Campbell, 2001; Ussher et al., 2012). Even women from conservative societies living in developed countries like Australia are seen to be discouraged by family to obtain information on sex and sexual health risks before marriage (Meldrum et al., 2016). Therefore, women who have a conservative sociocultural background are believed to be at risk of HIV/STIs because either they do not have enough information about sexual health risks or they are not encouraged to negotiate safer sex with husbands/partners, even while being aware that husbands/partners may have concurrent sexual partnerships (Parikh, 2007).

Gay men may sometimes engage in sexual risk-taking, even being aware of the risk of HIV/STIs. Often, family rejection of gay men's sexual identity is seen to compel them to seek support from peers (Fauk et al., 2017). While peers can provide social support without being judgmental of diverse sexual/gender identities, engagement in gay communities can sometimes lead to sexual risk-taking (Muriuki et al., 2011). Green (2008), for instance, in his study of gay men in the United States, shows that sometimes gay men who have more erotic capital, being tall and athletic, are most valued in the sexual field – a social space where gay men congregate to fulfil their erotic appetites. Therefore, gay men who have less erotic capital might struggle to establish ties with other gay men who may propose to have condomless sex. Therefore, researchers like Wilkerson et al. (2010) suggest that sexual risk-taking may become necessary when less experienced gay men struggle to gain acceptance in gay communities.

Other researchers, notably those who explored intimate partnerships among gay men, found that gay intimate partners believe that sex without condoms can be a sign of trust and commitment and that condom use means rejection of a sexual partner (Donovan et al., 1994; Prieur, 1990). Therefore, Donovan et al. (1994) argue that in intimate partnerships, for gay men, sex without using condoms can be 'an expression of positive values and good feelings' (p. 613).

Trust, intimacy, and loyalty are important qualities to sustain an intimate relationship. Taggart et al. (2017) suggest that intimate partners may not use condoms due to their belief that condom use represents mistrust in primary relationships and that not using condoms can build intimacy and closeness. This scenario was evident in a study of HYP in the United States, who reported not using condoms with intimate partners, even being cognisant of sexual health risks, as they believed that negotiating condom use with a primary partner might lead to questions about loyalty (Wagner et al., 2001).

Engagement in paid sex may also impact condom use. Studies from developing countries emphasise poverty: sex workers may offer condomless sex and charge more for it (Dunn et al., 2017; Mahapatra et al., 2013; Wojcicki & Malala, 2001). Researchers like Poteat et al. (2015) suggest that in countries where sex work is illegal, police often use *possession of condoms* as evidence of sex work, and this can hinder sex workers to use condoms with clients all the times. There is also evidence of how, in some developing countries like India, policemen may coerce sex workers to have sex with them (Chakrapani et al., 2007; Mayhew et al., 2009). For instance, Chakrapani et al. (2007), in their study from India, found that sex workers reported that policemen sometimes took male sex workers to the police station and raped them, which presented the risk of HIV/STIs.

Overall, studies reviewed in this section show how structural and contextual forces may operate to shape young people's sexual behaviour. Notably, studies suggest that structural forces like poverty, patriarchy, and heteronormativity can produce contexts in which young people may not ensure sexual safety, even while being aware of the risk of HIV/STIs.

Conclusion

In this chapter, I have reviewed studies concerning young people's sex- and HIV/STI-related beliefs and factors that may shape those beliefs as well as their sexual behaviour. Broadly speaking, the review suggests that social structural forces, notably religion and heteronormativity, which produce beliefs regarding sex and HIV/STIs, may also constrain an individual's sexual behaviour. For instance, on the one hand, religion, patriarchy, and heteronormativity link sex outside marriage and same-sex sex with morality, enforcing the belief that such acts are the root causes of HIV/STIs. On the other hand, these structures constrain young people in their ability to negotiate safer sex with partners.

The few studies from Pakistan generally highlight the relationship between young people's knowledge about STIs and their sexual practices. However, these studies do not address social structural forces that may shape young people's sexual behaviour. Taking this study gap and conclusions drawn from the review above into consideration, I suggest that the theory of capital and social practice (Bourdieu, 1984 [1979], 1986) is well suited to identify linkages between young people's knowledge regarding HIV/STIs, structural and contextual constraints, and sexual behaviour. Notably, the theory can uncover this relationship by helping to analyse how limited social and financial capital may play out in shaping HYP's worldview that they have limited opportunities to survive and that negotiating sexual safety with primary/casual partners may impede their access to the limited social and financial support available at their disposal.

References

Abrar, N., & Ghouri, A. M. (2010). AIDS/HIV knowledge, attitude and beliefs of adolescents of Pakistan. *European Journal of Social Sciences, 16*(2), 275–285.

Adamczyk, A., & Hayes, B. E. (2012). Religion and sexual behaviors: Understanding the influence of Islamic cultures and religious affiliation for explaining sex outside of marriage. *American Sociological Review, 77*(5), 723–746.

Addai, I. (2000). Religious affiliation and sexual initiation among Ghanaian women. *Review of Religious Research, 41*(3), 328–343.

Agha, S. (2009). Changes in the timing of sexual initiation among young Muslim and Christian women in Nigeria. *Archives of Sexual Behavior, 38*(6), 899–908.

Andrinopoulos, K., Figueroa, J. P., Kerrigan, D., & Ellen, J. M. (2011). Homophobia, stigma and HIV in Jamaican prisons. *Culture, Health & Sexuality, 13*(2), 187–200.

Bello, A. H. (2011). The punishment for adultery in Islamic law and its application in Nigeria. *Journal of Islamic Law and Culture, 13*(2–3), 166–182.

Bourdieu, P. (1984 [1979]). *Distinction: A social critique of the judgment of taste.* Harvard University Press.

Bourdieu, P. (1986). The forms of capital. In J. G. Richardson (Ed.), *Handbook of theory and research for the sociology* (pp. 241–258). Greenwood.

Byron, P. (2017). Friendship, sexual intimacy and young people's negotiations of sexual health. *Culture, Health & Sexuality, 19*(4), 486–500.

Chakrapani, V., Newman, P. A., Shunmugam, M., McLuckie, A., & Melwin, F. (2007). Structural violence against Kothi–identified men who have sex with men in Chennai, India: A qualitative investigation. *AIDS Education & Prevention, 19*(4), 346–364.

Conner, M., & Norman, P. (2015). Predicting and changing health behavior: A social cognition approach. In M. Conner & P. Norman (Eds.), *Predicting and changing health behaviour: research and practice with social cognition models.* Open University Press.

Cowan, F., & Bell, G. (2011). STI control and prevention. In K. E. Rogstad (Ed.), *ABC of sexually transmitted infections.* Blackwell Publishing Limited.

Delobelle, P., Onya, H., Langa, C., Mashamba, J., & Depoorter, A. M. (2010). Advances in health promotion in Africa: Promoting health through hospitals. *Global Health Promotion, 17*(2 Suppl), 33–36.

Donovan, C., Mearns, C., McEwan, R., & Sugden, R. (1994). A review of the HIV-related sexual behaviour of gay men and men who have sex with men. *AIDS Care, 6*(5), 605–617.

Dunn, J., Zhang, Q., Weeks, M. R., Li, J., Liao, S., & Li, F. (2017). Indigenous HIV prevention beliefs and practices among low-earning Chinese sex workers as context for introducing female condoms and other novel prevention options. *Qualitative Health Research, 27*(9), 1302–1315.

Fauk, N. K., Merry, M. S., Sigilipoe, M. A., Putra, S., & Mwanri, L. (2017). Culture, social networks and HIV vulnerability among men who have sex with men in Indonesia. *PLoS One, 12*(6), e0178736.

Finke, R., & Adamczyk, A. (2008). Explaining morality: Using international data to reestablish the macro/micro link. *Sociological Quarterly, 49*(4), 617–652.

Fonner, V. A., Dalglish, S. L., Kennedy, C. E., Baggaley, R., O'reilly, K. R., Koechlin, F. M., ... Grant, R. M. (2016). Effectiveness and safety of oral HIV preexposure prophylaxis for all populations. *AIDS (London, England), 30*(12), 1973.

Ford, N., Migone, C., Calmy, A., Kerschberger, B., Kanters, S., Nsanzimana, S., ... Shubber, Z. (2018). Benefits and risks of rapid initiation of antiretroviral therapy. *AIDS, 32*(1), 17–23.

Foucault, M. (1990). *The history of sexuality: An introduction.* Vintage.

Garofalo, R., Kuhns, L. M., Hidalgo, M., Gayles, T., Kwon, S., Muldoon, A. L., & Mustanski, B. (2015). Impact of religiosity on the sexual risk behaviors of young men who have sex with men. *Journal of Sex Research, 52*(2), 590–598.

Gebhardt, W. A., Van Empele, P., & Van Beurden, D. (2009). Predicting preparatory behaviours for condom use in female undergraduate students: A one-year follow-up study. *International Journal of STD & AIDS, 20*(3), 161–164.

Gillmore, M. R., Archibald, M. E., Morrison, D. M., Wilsdon, A., Wells, E. A., Hoppe, M. J., ... Murowchick, E. (2002). Teen sexual behavior: Applicability of the theory of reasoned action. *Journal of Marriage & Family, 64*(4), 885–897.

Green, A. I. (2008). The social organization of desire: The sexual fields approach. *Sociological Theory, 26*(1), 25–50.

Gross, G., & Tyring, S. K. (2011). *Sexually transmitted infections and sexually transmitted diseases.* Springer.

Hamid, S., Johansson, E., & Rubenson, B. (2010). Security lies in obedience-voices of young women of a slum in Pakistan. *BMC Public Health, 10*(1), 164.

Henshaw, A. L. (2014). Geographies of tolerance: Human development, heteronormativity, and religion. *Sexuality & Culture, 18*(4), 959–976.

Herz, M., & Johansson, T. (2015). The normativity of the concept of heteronormativity. *Journal of Homosexuality, 62*(8), 1009–1020.

Kang, E., Delzell, D. A., & Mbonyingabo, C. (2017). Understanding HIV transmission and illness stigma: A relationship revisited in rural Rwanda. *AIDS Education and Prevention, 29*(6), 540–553.

Kasprzyk, D., Montaño, D. E., & Fishbein, M. (1998). Application of an integrated behavioral model to predict condom use: A prospective study among high HIV risk groups. *Journal of Applied Social Psychology, 28*(17), 1557–1583.

Kippax, S., Stephenson, N., Parker, R. G., & Aggleton, P. (2013). Between individual agency and structure in HIV prevention: Understanding the middle ground of social practice. *American Journal of Public Health, 103*(8), 1367–1375.

Liamputtong, P. (2013). Stigma, discrimination, and HIV/AIDS: An introduction. In *Stigma, discrimination and living with HIV/AIDS* (pp. 1–19). Springer.

Longfield, K., Cramer, R., & Sachingongu, N. (2003). *Misconceptions, folk beliefs, & denial: Young men's risk for STIs & HIV/AIDS in Zambia.* Retrieved from https://www.psi.org/wp-content/uploads/2003/10/WP53.pdf

MacPhail, C., & Campbell, C. (2001). 'I think condoms are good but, aai, I hate those things': Condom use among adolescents and young people in a Southern African township. *Social Science & Medicine, 52*(11), 1613–1627.

Mahapatra, B., Lowndes, C. M., Mohanty, S. K., Gurav, K., Ramesh, B. M., Moses, S., ... Alary, M. (2013). Factors associated with risky sexual practices among female sex workers in Karnataka, India. *PLoS One, 8*(4), e62167.

Maulana, A. O., Krumeich, A., & Van Den Borne, B. (2009). Emerging discourse: Islamic teaching in HIV prevention in Kenya. *Culture, Health & Sexuality, 11*(5), 559–569.

Mayhew, S., Collumbien, M., Qureshi, A., Platt, L., Rafiq, N., Faisel, A., ... Hawkes, S. (2009). Protecting the unprotected: Mixed-method research on drug use, sex work and rights in Pakistan's fight against HIV/AIDS. *Sexually Transmitted Infections, 85*(Suppl 2), ii31–ii36.

Meldrum, R., Liamputtong, P., & Wollersheim, D. (2014). Caught between two worlds: Sexuality and young Muslim women in Melbourne, Australia. *Sexuality & Culture, 18*(1), 166–179.

Meldrum, R. M., Liamputtong, P., & Wollersheim, D. (2016). Sexual health knowledge and needs: Young Muslim women in Melbourne, Australia. *International Journal of Health Services, 46*(1), 124–140.

Menon, J. A., Thankian, K., & Mwaba, S. O. (2015). Impact of information leaflet on human immunodeficiency virus (HIV) related information and self management in HIV positive adolescents. *Journal of AIDS and HIV Research, 7*(5), 55–60.

Mmari, K., Kalamar, A. M., Brahmbhatt, H., & Venables, E. (2016). The influence of the family on adolescent sexual experience: A comparison between Baltimore and Johannesburg. *PLoS One, 11*(11), e0166032.

Montanaro, E. A., & Bryan, A. D. (2014). Comparing theory-based condom interventions: Health belief model versus theory of planned behavior. *Health Psychology, 33*(10), 1251–1260.

Mshana, G., Plummer, M. L., Wamoyi, J., Shigongo, Z. S., Ross, D. A., & Wight, D. (2006). 'She was bewitched and caught an illness similar to AIDS': AIDS and sexually transmitted infection causation beliefs in rural northern Tanzania. *Culture, Health & Sexuality, 8*(1), 45–58.

Muriuki, A. M., Fendrich, M., Pollack, L. M., & Lippert, A. M. (2011). Civic participation and risky sexual behavior among urban US men who have sex with men. *Journal of HIV/AIDS & Social Services, 10*(4), 376–394.

Mutonyi, H., Nashon, S., & Nielsen, W. S. (2010). Perceptual influence of Ugandan biology students' understanding of HIV/AIDS. *Research in Science Education, 40*(4), 573–588.

NACP. (2014). *Global AIDS response progress report 2014: Country progress report Pakistan.* Retrieved from http://nacp.gov.pk/repository/howwework/Publications/GARPR%202014.pdf

Nicoll, A., Laukamm-Josten, U., Mwizarubi, B., Mayala, C., Mkuye, M., Nyembela, G., & Grosskurth, H. (1993). Lay health beliefs concerning HIV and AIDS—A barrier for control programmes. *AIDS Care, 5*(2), 231–241.

Nleya, P. T., & Segale, E. (2015). How Setswana cultural beliefs and practices on sexuality affect teachers' and adolescents' sexual decisions, practices, and experiences as well as HIV/aids and STI prevention in select Botswanan secondary schools. *Journal of the International Association of Providers of AIDS Care (JIAPAC), 14*(3), 224–233.

Nuwaha, F., Faxelid, E., Neema, S., & Höjer, B. (2001). Lay people's perceptions of sexually transmitted infections in Uganda. *International Journal of STD & AIDS, 10*(11), 709–717.

Oluduro, O. (2010). The role of religious leaders in curbing the spread of HIV/AIDS in Nigeria. *Potchefstroom Electronic Law Journal/Potchefstroomse Elektroniese Regsblad, 13*(3), 208–236.

Parikh, S. A. (2007). The political economy of marriage and HIV: The ABC approach, "safe" infidelity, and managing moral risk in Uganda. *American Journal of Public Health, 97*(7), 198–1208.

Poteat, T., Wirtz, A. L., Radix, A., Borquez, A., Silva-Santisteban, A., Deutsch, M. B., … Operario, D. (2015). HIV risk and preventive interventions in transgender women sex workers. *The Lancet, 385*(9964), 274–286.

Prieur, A. (1990). Norwegian gay men: Reasons for continued practice of unsafe sex. *AIDS Education and Prevention, 2*(2), 109–115.

Qadir, F., de Silva, P., Prince, M., & Khan, M. (2005). Marital satisfaction in Pakistan: A pilot investigation. *Sexual and Relationship Therapy, 20*(2), 195–209.

Raheel, H., White, F., Kadir, M. M., & Fatmi, Z. (2007). Knowledge and beliefs of adolescents regarding sexually transmitted infections and HIV/AIDS in a rural district in Pakistan. *Journal of the Pakistan Medical Association, 57*(1), 8–11.

Rajabali, A., Khan, S., Warraich, H. J., Khanani, M. R., & Ali, S. H. (2008). HIV and homosexuality in Pakistan. *Infectious Diseases, 8*(8), 511–515.

Raza, M. I., Afifi, A., Choudhry, A. J., & Khan, H. I. (1998). Knowledge, attitude and behaviour towards AIDS among educated youth in Lahore, Pakistan. *Journal of the Pakistan Medical Association, 48*, 179–181.

Sheeran, P., & Taylor, S. (1999). Predicting intentions to use condoms: A meta-analysis and comparison of the theories of reasoned action and planned behavior. *Journal of Applied Social Psychology, 29*(8), 1624–1675.

Taggart, T., Ellen, J., & Arrington-Sanders, R. (2017). Young African American male–male relationships: Experiences, expectations, and condom use. *Journal of LGBT Youth, 14*(4), 80–392.

Taylor, D., Bury, M., Campling, N., Carter, S., Garfied, S., Newbould, J., & Rennie, T. (2006). *A review of the use of the Health Belief Model (HBM), the Theory of Reasoned Action (TRA), the Theory of Planned Behaviour (TPB) and the Trans-Theoretical Model (TTM) to study and predict health related behaviour change.* Retrieved from https://www.researchgate.net/profile/Timothy-Rennie/publication/334114235_A_Review_of_the_use_of_the_Health_Belief_Model_HBM_the_Theory_of_Reasoned_Action_TRA_the_Theory_of_Planned_Behaviour_TPB_and_the_Trans-Theoretical_Model_TTM_to_study_and_predict_health_related_behavio/links/5d17a5d8299bf1547c8927c4/A-Review-of-the-use-of-the-Health-Belief-Model-HBM-the-Theory-of-Reasoned-Action-TRA-the-Theory-of-Planned-Behaviour-TPB-and-the-Trans-Theoretical-Model-TTM-to-study-and-predict-health-related-behav.pdf

Tyson, M., Covey, J., & Rosenthal, H. E. (2014). Theory of planned behavior interventions for reducing heterosexual risk behaviors: A meta-analysis. *Health Psychology, 33*(12), 1454–1467.

UNAIDS. (2018). *Global HIV & AIDS statistics – 2018 fact sheet.* Retrieved from http://www.unaids.org/sites/default/files/media_asset/UNAIDS_FactSheet_en.pdf

Ussher, J. M., Rhyder-Obid, M., Perz, J., Rae, M., Wong, T. W., & Newman, P. (2012). Purity, privacy and procreation: Constructions and experiences of sexual and reproductive health in Assyrian and Karen women living in Australia. *Sexuality & Culture, 16*(4), 467–485.

Vanlandingham, M. J., Suprasert, S., Grandjean, N., & Sittitrai, W. (1995). Two views of risky sexual practices among northern Thai males: The health belief model and the theory of reasoned action. *Journal of Health and Social Behavior, 36*(2), 95–212.

Villarruel, A. M., Jemmott, J. B., Jemmott, L. S., & Ronis, D. L. (2004). Predictors of sexual intercourse and condom use intentions among Spanish-dominant Latino youth: A test of the planned behavior theory. *Nursing Research, 53*(3), 172–181.

Von Haeften, I., & Kensk, K. (2001). Multi-partnered heterosexuals' condom use for vaginal sex with their main partner as a function of attitude, subjective norm, partner norm, perceived behavioural control and weighted control beliefs. *Psychology, Health & Medicine, 6*(2), 165–177.

Wagner, L. S., Carlin, L., Cauce, A. M., & Tenner, A. (2001). A snapshot of homeless youth in Seattle: Their characteristics, behaviors and beliefs about HIV protective strategies. *Journal of Community Health, 26*(1), 219–223.

Warwick, I., Aggleton, P., & Homans, H. (1988). Constructing commonsense—Young people's beliefs about AIDS. *Sociology of Health & Illness, 10*(3), 213–233.

Widman, L., Golin, C. E., Grodensky, C. A., & Suchindran, C. (2013). Do safer sex self-efficacy, attitudes toward condoms, and HIV transmission risk beliefs differ among men who have sex with men, heterosexual men, and women living with HIV? *AIDS and Behavior, 17*(5), 1873–1882.

Wilkerson, J. M., Brooks, A. K., & Ross, M. W. (2010). Sociosexual identity development and sexual risk taking of acculturating collegiate gay and bisexual men. *Journal of College Student Development, 51*(3), 279–296.

Williams, I., Daniels, D., Gedela, K., Briggs, A., & Pryce, A. (2011). HIV. In K. E. Rogstad (Ed.), *ABC of sexually transmitted infections.* Blackwell Publishing Limited.

Wojcicki, J. M., & Malala, J. (2001). Condom use, power and HIV/AIDS risk: Sex-workers bargain for survival in Hillbrow/Joubert Park/Berea, Johannesburg. *Social Science & Medicine, 53*(1), 99–121.

Wulfert, E., & Wan, C. K. (1995). Safer sex intentions and condom use viewed from a health belief, reasoned action, and social cognitive perspective. *Journal of Sex Research, 32*(4), 299–311.

Chapter 4
The Theory of Capital and Social Practice

Chapters 2 and 3 demonstrate how previous research has shown that a combination of social structural and interpersonal forces can shape young people's homelessness, their street-related experiences, and sexual behaviour. For instance, studies reviewed in Chap. 2 show how homelessness is produced as a result of interactions between structural and individual-level issues. Similarly, studies reviewed in Chap. 3 show that structural forces that influence beliefs regarding sex and HIV and sexually transmitted infections (STIs) can also constrain individuals' sexual behaviour. In developing a study that can examine the relationships between various social structural- and interpersonal-level forces, it is critical to draw on a social theory that has a *relational* view of social practice. Therefore, the theoretical framework adopted in the present study is based on the constructivist sociology of Pierre Bourdieu (1984 [1979], 1986, 1989). Because Bourdieu's theory of capital and social practice posits that social structure and social practice are mutually constitutive, it can elucidate how homeless young people's (HYP's) socially disadvantaged position contributes to their sexual risk-taking, thereby increasing their risk of HIV/STIs.

This chapter comprises four sections. The first section describes the main tenets of Bourdieusian theory, including how the interrelationship between social fields, habitus, and capital produces social practice. The second section provides a detailed description of social fields, which are social spaces in which individuals navigate their social lives by accumulating and deploying various forms of capital. The third section describes habitus: individuals' long-lasting dispositions structured by their past and present experiences, which also orient their behaviour in specific contexts. The fourth section discusses the forms of capital: financial, social, and cultural resources that individuals accumulate and deploy to improve their social and/or financial status in a given social field. The chapter closes by describing how the concepts of social fields, habitus, and capital are used to analyse and explain the results of the present study.

M. N. Noor, *Homeless Youth of Pakistan*, SpringerBriefs in Public Health, https://doi.org/10.1007/978-3-030-79305-0_4

A Relational View of Social Practice

Bourdieu's theory posits that society is a multidimensional space of social relations called *social fields* (Bourdieu & Wacquant, 1992). The economy, education, arts, bureaucracy, and politics are various examples of social fields. Within social fields, individuals are placed in a social hierarchy based on their *habitus* (i.e. a combination of dispositions, competencies, and worldviews) and the unique configuration of *capital* they possess (i.e. a combination of economic, social, and cultural resources). Individuals' social practices are shaped by the interaction between a given social field, their habitus, and the forms of capital they possess. While social fields are spaces that offer individuals opportunities to navigate their social lives, habitus enables individuals to recognise the boundaries of, and their relative positions within, a given social field. A unique property of social fields is their internal logic, which Bourdieu (1990, p. 68) refers to as *doxa* that, through individuals' habitus, gives them a sense of their legitimate position in relation to others. Bourdieu (1986) attempts to move away from the materialist conception of power and social inequality by arguing that capital can exist in three fundamental forms that include economic, social, and cultural capital. Importantly, he links forms of capital with the dynamics of a given social field, such that accruing specific forms of capital that are valued in a given field would be critical to individuals' improvement of their socioeconomic status.

While it is important to examine how social field, habitus, and capital are interdependent and interact to produce social practice or a social phenomenon, it is also critical to understand the specific function each component plays in social reproduction. The following sections attempt to deconstruct the concepts of social fields, habitus, and capital, in turn.

Social Fields

Bourdieu's concept of social field can be thought of as a 'football field', a bordered space consisting of positions occupied by players who draw on specific skills to play the football game, controlled by certain rules. There are limits to how the game can be played within a football field, the conditions of which can differ: 'wet, dry, grass or full of potholes' (Thomson, 2008, p. 69). Bourdieu also views social life as a game where individuals play in the social world – a broader field of power that consists of various social fields or spaces like economic, educational, bureaucratic, or political fields. Because social fields are numerous and are activity-specific, they have their histories, rules, and stakes. However, unlike a football field, a social field is not a level playing field, as individuals have unique habitus and forms of capital (discussed in more detail in the following sections).

For Bourdieu (1998), a social field is a structured space of hierarchical social relationships produced through the unequal distribution of financial and cultural resources:

A structured social space, a field of forces, a force field. It contains people who dominate and people who are dominated. Constant, permanent relationships of inequality operate inside this space, which at the same becomes a space in which various actors struggle for the transformation of or preservation of the field. All the individuals in this universe bring to the competition all the (relative) power at their disposal. It is this power that defines their position in the field and, as a result, their strategies. (Bourdieu, 1998, p. 40)

In other words, social fields are structured spaces that facilitate, order, and constrain human activity. To navigate their social lives, individuals follow patterns, regularities, or rules, which Bourdieu refers to as doxa. The doxa controls individuals by making their social practices somewhat predictable, without which society would become anarchic (Thomson, 2008). Importantly, each field is socially constructed, has a unique history of development, enables specific activities, and thereby has distinct doxa, the 'logic of practice' (Bourdieu, 1990, p. 80). The doxa enables individuals who occupy specific positions to understand how to act within a given social field (Shammas & Sandberg, 2015).

Another important aspect of Bourdieu's concept of social fields is that social fields are connected through relationships of exchange. For instance, the kind of schooling individuals receive in the educational field can determine how they are positioned in the formal job market. Moreover, social fields are also placed at a hierarchy within the field of power: the dominant fields can shape the dynamics of other fields. For example, the conditions of the housing field are very much dependent on the conditions of the political (the state) and economic fields.

In recent years, some researchers have employed the concept of social fields to understand mechanisms that lead to the formation of the street culture and its internal dynamics, specifically in developed world setting (Barker, 2016; Bryant, 2018; Green, 2008; Shammas & Sandberg, 2015). For instance, Shammas and Sandberg (2015) conceptualise how the existence of drug dealing culture, which they call the *street field*, may be produced and reinforced by the conditions of the states' economic, political, bureaucratic, and legal fields. Notably, they describe how the economic recession, the stigmatising effects of a criminal record, and racial discrimination can contribute to an increased concentration of young people on the streets, whose financial gains may be contingent on practices like panhandling, theft, and drug dealing. Barker (2013), however, emphasises how various forms of capital play out in the formation and function of the *field of homeless young people* (p. 361). He suggests that since HYP's lives are characterised by the lack of economic and social capital, the field can provide them with opportunities to survive in adverse social conditions. Violence and crime, which Barker (2013) considers a form of *cultural capital*, is most valued in the field since it helps young people to gain some material benefits as well as gives them a sense of autonomy, self-identity, and empowerment.

These studies provide important insights into how the street-based social field acts as a gateway to various opportunities – however unorthodox – to accumulate material and social resources. There is a dearth of research that employs the concept of social field to understand street-based sexual experiences. Green (2008) comes close, however, in using the concept of *sexual fields* (p. 26) to explain the dynamics of gay communities in the United States. His conceptualisation of sexual fields represents a social space where gay men congregate to socialise and to satisfy their erotic appetites. He further elaborates that in the sexual fields, *erotic capital* (p. 27) is the most valued form of capital. For instance, being a gay man with a tall and muscular build would increase one's value as a sexual partner in gay clubs. In contrast, any man who was not tall and/or athletic would incur a capital deficit, contributing to his structural disadvantage within the field. The *capital deficit* (p. 41) can lead gay men to engage 'in unprotected anal intercourse as strategic compensation for low status or because of reduced power to set sexual limits on the exchange' (p. 43).

Habitus

Bourdieu's concept of *habitus* cannot be straightforwardly explained: it 'can be both revelatory and mystifying, instantly recognizable and difficult to define, straightforward and slippery' (Manton, 2008, p. 49). In society, individuals may assume that they are 'free agents' who make choices and decisions following the slightly predictable behaviour of others. The concept of habitus helps us to examine how those choices and decisions are shaped by regularities that exist in society and makes it possible to explain the relationship between social structure and individual agency, and the social mechanisms through which the 'outer "social", and "inner" self, help to shape each other' (Manton, 2008, p. 50).

Bourdieu (1990) defines habitus as a *system* of dispositions available to an individual based on their social experiences and history, which orient their actions in various situations. Habitus is a property of social agents, which include individuals, groups, or social fields. It is a system of dispositions, which is systematically structured rather than being randomly patterned (Pickel, 2005). Habitus is *structured* in that it is shaped by individuals' past conditions of existence. It, at the same time, is *structuring* because it shapes individuals' present and future practices (Collyer et al., 2015).

The term *disposition* is critical to Bourdieu's concept of habitus in bringing structure and agency together. Dispositions can be understood as individuals' propensities that shape their choices, decisions, and behaviours, which can often reflect the structure of social fields that are constitutive of their habitus. Dispositions are 'durable in that they last over time and transposable in being capable of becoming active within a wide variety of theatres of social life' (Manton, 2008, p. 51). So, if defined less formally, habitus can be understood as individuals' *worldviews* and their ways of thinking, perceiving, or responding in different social situations, and it also depicts how individuals' actions and choices are shaped by their histories.

Using the concept of habitus, some scholars have attempted to explain specific behaviours of homeless and other disadvantaged young people in the context of the developed world (Bryant, 2018; Fraser, 2013; Shammas & Sandberg, 2015; Wacquant, 2002). Wacquant (2002) was the first to introduce the concept of the *street habitus* to examine the entrenchment of African American homeless people in the street culture of panhandling, scavenging, violence, and drug use/dealing. Reflecting on the stories of some homeless men who failed to retain jobs in the formal market and returned to street life, Wacquant (2002) suggested that their conduct could be better understood in terms of the effects of their previous socialisation on the streets. Bourgois and Schonberg (2007), however, highlight the ethnic dimension of African American homeless people. Their concept of *ethnicised habitus* (p. 7) represents how ethnic discrimination embedded in political, economic, and ideological domains in the United States contributes to the marginalisation of African Americans and shapes their participation in gangs, violence, and drug use/dealing. In addition, Barker (2016) has pointed to another dimension of habitus, the *habitus of instability* (p. 671), while explaining how homelessness is reinforced among young people living in Australia. The concept of the habitus of instability represents how HYP internalise a sense of insecurity and instability through their experiences of familial disruption, joblessness, and unstable living conditions. These internalised dispositions may give young people a *sense of their place in the world* (Bryant, 2018, p. 987), characterised by the view that their circumstances will remain unchanged, which entrenches them in the street life.

While Wacquant's (2002) street habitus emphasises how homeless people's engagement in street culture can create a disjuncture between dispositions they acquire from it (i.e. inclination to commit aggression, violence, and drug use/dealing) and conventional social life, Bourgois and Schonberg's (2007) ethnicised habitus reveals how racial discrimination can play out in shaping homeless people's perception about their social disadvantage. Barker's (2016) habitus of instability explains how past and ongoing experiences of instability can lead HYP to anticipate that their status of instability would be intractable. Although these researchers discuss distinct dimensions of HYP's habitus, there are some common elements: dispositions are durable, they are based on past and present experiences, and they shape future practices.

Forms of Capital

Bourdieu (1986) describes capital as resources that individuals possess. He suggests that there are three basic forms of capital: economic, cultural, and social. However, other scholars have advanced Bourdieu's work by introducing the concepts of negative social and cultural capital; formal, informal, horizontal, and vertical social capital; cultural health capital; and erotic capital, through the empirical application, turning them into sophisticated tools for analysing social reproduction and mobility (Barker, 2013; Green, 2008; Hakim, 2010; Shim, 2010; Wacquant, 1998; Warr, 2005).

Economic capital can be understood as individuals' income, monetary assets, and different financial resources institutionalised in the form of property rights (Bourdieu, 1986). Economic capital is most valued among individuals across various social fields and makes possible access to different opportunities, permitting individuals to accumulate more wealth and power (English & Bolton, 2016).

Bourdieu (1986) posits that economic capital can be accumulated most easily and can easily be transferred from one person to another. It can also be easily converted into cultural and social capital. For instance, economic capital is converted into cultural and social capital when a person pays school fees to attain an education, which can be mobilized to secure a higher-paying job.

Cultural capital refers to embodied assets such as knowledge, values, attitudes, or tastes (Bourdieu, 1986). Cultural capital is further classified into three forms: *embodied, institutionalised,* and *objectified.* Embodied cultural capital refers to individuals' cultural knowledge (i.e. etiquette, mannerisms, language, values, or norms) that guides their social behaviours. Institutionalised cultural capital can be understood as individuals' educational qualifications; to accumulate it, individuals are required to go through a formal process (i.e. examination) and obtain a certificate of competence (i.e. diploma, degree) that differentiates them from a self-taught person. Objectified cultural capital can be described as different cultural goods such as books, paintings, or machines that individuals produce or acquire by using embodied as well as institutionalised cultural capital. According to Bourdieu (1986), the properties of objectified cultural capital can be better described by considering its relationship with embodied cultural capital. Ownership and transmissibility of objectified cultural capital are important: objectified cultural capital can be possessed both materially and symbolically in so far as that owning a book presupposes economic capital, while writing a book presupposes embodied and institutionalised cultural capital. This indicates that legal ownership of the objectified cultural capital is transmissible in terms of its materiality. However, the symbolic capital that is fundamentally a precondition to produce objectified cultural capital is not transmissible.

Some scholars have applied the concept of cultural capital to particularly understand how HYP acquire a repertoire of skills to survive on the streets and also how their actions are perceived by the general public (Barker, 2013; Sandberg, 2008; Shammas & Sandberg, 2015). In particular, Shammas and Sandberg (2015) introduce the concept of *street capital* (p. 206) to explain a range of material resources and practices among street-based drug dealers. They conceptualised the street capital as a combination of three distinct but interrelated components: a dispositional form – an understanding of what *crimes* are legitimate in the street field, and the use of violence and drugs; an objectified form – the possession of material things like weapons and drugs; and an institutionalised form – their recognition as criminals based on their official criminal record. Barker (2013), in his research with Australian HYP, used the term *negative cultural capital* (p. 361), borrowed from Wacquant (1998) to explain how the use of violence and drugs is perceived within and outside the street field. He suggested that while the use of violence and drugs is a means for young people to take control of their lives, to obtain physical protection, and to accrue social and material capital, these practices are perceived negatively or as counterproductive by the general public, which can reinforce young people's marginalisation. This empirical work further suggests that forms of capital are field-specific, and their value is dependent on their relationship to the given fields. For instance, the use of violence and drugs has value in the street field but is viewed as pathological and dangerous in mainstream fields such as legal, educational, and bureaucratic.

The concept of *social capital* can be dated back to 1916 when Hanifan introduced the concept of community social capital (p. 131) in *The rural school community centre*. Adopting a micro-level approach, Hanifan (1916) highlighted how social connectedness can benefit individuals in a given community. Later, scholars like Bourdieu (1986), Coleman (1988), and Putnam (1993) reconceptualised social capital in their effort to foreground the importance of strong social ties that can facilitate productive social actions. In these explanations, social closeness, trust, obligations, and reciprocity were considered important elements that strengthen social ties. Putnam (1993) developed two important dimensions of social capital: bonding and bridging social capital. Bonding networks refer to *horizontal ties* where people are intimately or emotionally connected with each other, such as family, relatives, friends, or even neighbourhood ties. Bridging networks represent *vertical ties*, which may connect people across diverse social divisions based on gender, ethnicity, age, and social class (Warr, 2005, p. 286). Szreter and Woolcock (2004) suggest an important variation of bridging networks – the *linking social capital* – which refers to connections among individuals who are unequal in terms of social status and power. This social capital intends to make a connection between communities, societies, or even the states.

Similar to theorisations of Coleman (1988) and Putnam (1993), Bourdieu's (1986) concept of social capital represents social networks as a resource for individuals. It is however important to note that Bourdieu's (1986) social capital is part of his broader theory that attempts to bridge the micro/macro dichotomy. Formally, Bourdieu (1986) describes social capital as

> the aggregate of the actual or potential resources which are linked to possession of a durable network of more or less institutionalized relationships of mutual acquaintance and recognition, or, in other words, to membership in a group – which provides each of its members with the backing of collectively-owned capital, a 'credential' which entitles them to credit, in the various senses of the word. (Bourdieu, 1986, p. 51)

Also, for Bourdieu (1986), social capital is *integrally linked* with other forms of capital, including economic and cultural capital. He describes how social capital can help individuals accumulate other forms of capital important to navigate social life in a given social field. For instance, for children, their families act as a source of social capital in that they can deploy economic capital (i.e. educational expenses) and connect them to educational networks, through which children can accumulate cultural capital (i.e. educational qualifications). Educational qualifications, in turn, can help individuals to connect to other sources of social capital (i.e. job networks) and economic capital (i.e. income generated through being part of a professional network).

Usually, studies describe how social capital, especially connections with informal and formal social networks, can help people to achieve personal goals (Lippman et al., 2018; Robertson et al., 2019; Wiltshire & Stevinson, 2018). Attempts have also been made to highlight the 'dark side' of social capital (Field, 2008, p. 89). For instance, Wacquant (1998) conceptualises the state as a source of *negative social capital*, specifically when the erosion of public services contributes to social inequality. He specifically describes how in the early 1970s, inefficient police protection and criminal justice systems and the deterioration of welfare, public health, and education services contributed to the marginalisation of the ghettos in Chicago. Barker (2012) describes the role of the family in shaping young people's life chances through the concept of social capital. He emphasises that for families, not being able to provide social and material support to young people can lead them to explore other options of support that can contribute to and reinforce their homelessness. Campbell (2001), in her research with a South African mining community, highlighted that the prevalence of HIV was higher among individuals connected with *savings clubs*, characterised by the increased alcohol consumption and sexual promiscuity, than individuals who were associated with religious and sports networks.

Recently, researchers like Green (2008) and Hakim (2010) have advanced Bourdieu's work by developing the concept of erotic capital. Hakim (2010) describes erotic capital as individuals' physical attributes that may act as a resource to help them to improve their social and financial status. Hakim (2010) suggests that erotic capital may be understood as a mixture of 'aesthetic, visual, physical, social, and sexual attractiveness to other members of your society, and especially to members of the opposite sex, in all social contexts' (p. 501). She further argues that erotic capital is a useful concept to understand the sexualised culture of the modern era. Elsewhere, in this chapter, I outlined how Green's (2008) empirical work in gay communities in the United States indicated the differential distribution of erotic capital in sexual fields – with black gay men, for example, being fetishised sexual partners in some gay clubs. Hakim (2010) further argues that erotic capital is often linked with economic, social, and cultural capital. For instance, she describes that while women do not usually have more erotic *power* than men, they have more erotic capital, meaning that women are more often displayed when it comes to commercial advertisements of products of all kinds. Moreover, she suggests that often attractive people who possess social skills are more likely to be successful in securing jobs.

Conclusion

This chapter describes the main tenets of Bourdieu's theory of capital and social practice, which helps to locate social processes that shape HYP's lives. The trio of social fields, habitus, and capital, and the various ways it has been developed through the empirical work of other scholars, can provide a lens to examine how the effect of structural forces, notably poverty, gender inequality, and sociosexual norms, can be translated into micro-level social encounters that contribute to young people's homelessness and their ongoing insecurity, which, in turn, shape their sexual choices, decisions, and practices.

References

Barker, J. D. (2012). Social capital, homeless young people and the family. *Journal of Youth Studies, 15*(6), 730–743.

Barker, J. D. (2013). Negative cultural capital and homeless young people. *Journal of Youth Studies, 16*(3), 358–374.

Barker, J. D. (2016). A habitus of instability: Youth homelessness and instability. *Journal of Youth Studies, 19*(5), 665–683.

Bourdieu, P. (1984 [1979]). *Distinction: A social critique of the judgment of taste.* Harvard University Press.

Bourdieu, P. (1986). The forms of capital. In J. G. Richardson (Ed.), *Handbook of theory and research for the sociology* (pp. 241–258). Greenwood.

Bourdieu, P. (1989). Social space and symbolic power. *Sociological Theory, 7*(1), 14–25.

Bourdieu, P. (1990). *The logic of practice* (N. Richard, Trans.). Stanford University Press.

Bourdieu, P. (1998). *On television* (P. P. Ferguson, Trans.). The New Press.

Bourdieu, P., & Wacquant, L. J. (1992). *An invitation to reflexive sociology.* University of Chicago Press.

Bourgois, P., & Schonberg, J. J. E. (2007). Intimate apartheid: Ethnic dimensions of habitus among homeless heroin injectors. *Ethnography, 8*(1), 7–31.

Bryant, J. (2018). Building inclusion, maintaining marginality: How social and health services act as capital for young substance users. *Journal of Youth Studies, 21*(7), 983–998.

Campbell, C. (2001). Social capital and health: Contextualising health promotion within local community networks. In S. Baron, J. Field, & T. Schuller (Eds.), *Social capital: Critical perspectives* (pp. 182–196). Oxford University Press.

Coleman, J. S. (1988). Social capital in the creation of human capital. *The American Journal of Sociology, 94*, S95–S120.

Collyer, F. M., Willis, K. F., Franklin, M., Harley, K., & Short, S. D. (2015). Healthcare choice: Bourdieu's capital, habitus and field. *Current Sociology, 63*(5), 685–699.

English, F. W., & Bolton, C. L. (2016). *Bourdieu for educators: Policy and practice.* SAGE Publications.

Field, J. (2008). *Social capital.* Routledge.

Fraser, A. (2013). Street habitus: Gangs, territorialism and social change in Glasgow. *Journal of Youth Studies, 16*(8), 970–985.

Green, A. I. (2008). The social organization of desire: The sexual fields approach. *Sociological Theory, 26*(1), 25–30.

Hakim, C. (2010). Erotic capital. *European Sociological Review, 26*(5), 499–518.

Hanifan, L. J. (1916). The rural school community center. *The Annals of the American Academy of Political and Social Science, 67*(1), 130–138.

Lippman, S. A., Leslie, H. H., Neilands, T. B., Twine, R., Grignon, J. S., MacPhail, C., … Kahn, K. (2018). Context matters: Community social cohesion and health behaviors in two South African areas. *Health and Place, 50*, 98–104.

Manton, K. (2008). Habitus. In M. Grenfell (Ed.), *Pierre Bourdieu: Key concepts* (pp. 49–65). Acumen Publishing Limited.

Pickel, A. (2005). The habitus process: A biopsychosocial conception. *Journal for the Theory of Social Behaviour, 35*, 437–461.

Putnam, R. D. (1993). The prosperous community. *The American Prospect, 4*(13), 35–42.

Robertson, J., Eime, R., & Westerbeek, H. (2019). Community sports clubs: Are they only about playing sport, or do they have broader health promotion and social responsibilities? *Annals of Leisure Research, 22*(2), 215–232.

Sandberg, S. (2008). Street capital, ethnicity and violence on the streets of Oslo. *Theoretical Criminology, 12*(2), 153–171.

Shammas, V. L., & Sandberg, S. (2015). Habitus, capital, and conflict: Bringing Bourdieusian field theory to criminology. *Criminology & Criminal Justice, 16*(2), 195–213.

Shim, J. K. (2010). Cultural health capital: A theoretical approach to understanding health care interactions and the dynamics of unequal treatment. *Journal of Health and Social Behavior, 51*(1), 1–15.

Szreter, S., & Woolcock, M. (2004). Health by association? Social capital, social theory, and the political economy of public health. *International Journal of Epidemiology, 33*(4), 650–667.

Thomson, P. (2008). Field. In M. Grenfell (Ed.), *Pierre Bourdieu: Key concepts* (pp. 67–81). Acumen Publishing Limited.

Wacquant, L. J. (1998). Negative social capital: State breakdown and social destitution in America's urban core. *Netherlands Journal of Housing and the Built Environment, 13*(1), 25.

Wacquant, L. J. (2002). Scrutinizing the street: Poverty, morality, and the pitfalls of urban ethnography. *American Journal of Sociology, 107*(6), 1468–1532.

Warr, D. J. (2005). Social networks in a 'discredited' neighbourhood. *Journal of Sociology, 41*(3), 285–308.

Wiltshire, G., & Stevinson, C. (2018). Exploring the role of social capital in community-based physical activity: Qualitative insights from parkrun. *Qualitative Research in Sport, Exercise and Health, 10*(1), 47–62. https://doi.org/10.1080/2159676X.2017.1376347

Chapter 5
Methodological Approach to the Study

The major aim of the present research is to examine the social processes shaping homeless young people's (HYP's) sexual practices that may put them at risk for HIV and other sexually transmitted infections (STIs). A cross-sectional qualitative approach was chosen as the way to fulfil this aim, as it facilitated an open exploration of HYP's views on their life chances and sexual experiences.

This chapter describes the methodological aspects of the research in three main sections. The first section outlines the study's ontological and epistemological assumptions. Based on the view that social reality is constructed through an interactional process of meaning-making, the research is underpinned by an idealist ontology and constructionist epistemology. In consonance with these philosophical assumptions, the abductive research strategy, which involves drawing on meanings and concepts that individuals give to their social experiences, was adopted. The second section describes the methods used to conduct the research. This section provides a detailed description of the study setting, HYP's selection criteria, the recruitment and interviewing process, and the data analysis method. The third section describes the key ethical considerations observed throughout the research journey: voluntary participation, the process of obtaining consent, and confidentiality. The chapter closes with a discussion on reflexivity regarding the research process, from my position as a partial 'insider' and 'outsider', and how this liminal positionality may have contributed to the conduct of the study in diverse ways.

Philosophical Starting Points

A social scientific enquiry is thought to begin with specific research paradigms, the broad philosophical and theoretical traditions within which attempts to understand the social world are conducted (Blaikie, 2007, p. 3). While a diverse range of

© The Author(s), under exclusive license to Springer Nature   39
Switzerland AG 2021
M. N. Noor, *Homeless Youth of Pakistan*, SpringerBriefs in Public Health,
https://doi.org/10.1007/978-3-030-79305-0_5

research paradigms such as positivism, social realism, critical rationalism, herme-neutics, ethnomethodology, critical theory, and social constructionism exist (Blaikie, 2007), researchers choose a specific approach based on their research objectives, personal beliefs, and professional socialisation. The present research is underpinned by the assumption that there is *no* single social *reality*, as it can be understood dif-ferently in different social contexts. Therefore, this study is underpinned by an ide-alist ontology and constructionist epistemology.

Ontological Assumptions

Ontology is concerned with the nature of reality and deals with the questions of 'what does exist as a reality, what it looks like, what units constitute it, and how these units interact with each other' (Blaikie, 2007, p. 3). Generally, realism and idealism represent two opposite poles of ontological assumptions. In its extreme form, realists believe that there is an objective reality existing independent of the human mind, which can be investigated using rigorous scientific methods. While shallow realists believe that reality is controlled by natural or social laws and can be observed through direct observation, conceptual realists emphasise rational think-ing rather than direct observation (Blaikie, 2007). Cautious realists, however, oppose these perspectives and hold that it is not possible to accurately perceive 'objective' reality due to imperfect human senses (Baehr, 1990).

Conversely, *idealists* reject the view that there exists an objective reality. Instead, they suggest that reality is socially constructed through an interactional process of meaning-making:

> In the *idealist* ontology, the external world consists of representations that are creations of individual minds. Whatever is regarded as being real is real only because we think it is real; it is simply an idea that has taken on the impression of being real. Reality is what human beings make or construct; it is the activities of creative subjects that constitute the world of objects. (Blaikie, 2007, p. 16)

The ontological assumption that underpins the present study aligns with that of idealism, which posits that social reality cannot be monistic but differs concerning the history and with specific sociocultural contexts. This view is also supported by the practice theory (Bourdieu, 1984 [1979], 1986) adopted in this study, which sug-gests that the social world is constructed through the interaction between social fields and the habitus of individuals. Therefore, I consider the study participants as the narrators of their social reality, produced through their interaction with other people as well as with structures like poverty, religion, sociosexual norms, patriar-chy, and heteronormativity.

Epistemological Assumptions

Epistemology is concerned with how social reality can be explored (Crotty, 1998). It provides researchers with a philosophical grounding upon which to make choices regarding research methods and justify their relevance and legitimacy. Blaikie (2007) defined epistemology as follows:

> Epistemology is concerned with the nature and scope of human knowledge, with what kinds of knowledge are possible, and with criteria for judging the adequacy of knowledge and for distinguishing between scientific and non-scientific knowledge. (Blaikie, 2007, p. 4)

Objectivism, subjectivism, and constructionism represent three distinct epistemological positions in philosophy (Blaikie, 2007). Objectivism is the view that there are intrinsic meanings attached to things in the world, and it is the researchers' responsibility to discover that meaning and that it is possible to do so. Subjectivism is the opposite of objectivism, with subjectivists assuming that 'things make no contribution to their meaning; the observer imposes it' (Hirst, 2011, p. 1). However, constructionism rejects both of them and posits that social reality is the product of a *meaning-giving activity* and depends on how people make sense of the social world around them (Blaikie, 2007, p. 22). For social constructionists, knowledge is a product of inter-subjective and meaning-giving activity between social actors and the researcher, and as Crotty (1998) argues,

> The focus of social constructionism is the collective generation and transmission of meaning. (Crotty, 1998, p. 58)

Also, constructionism is reflected in the practice theory (Bourdieu, 1984 [1979], 1986) adopted in this book, which suggests that the social world is constituted by a dialectical relationship between structure and human agency:

> On the one hand, the objective structures that the sociologist constructs, in the objectivist moment, by setting aside the subjective representations of the agents, form the basis for these representations and constitute the structural constraints that bear upon interactions; but, on the other hand, these representations must also be taken into consideration particularly if one wants to account for daily struggles, individual or collective, which purport to transform or to preserve these structures. This means that the two moments, the objectivist and subjectivist, stand in a dialectical relationship. (Bourdieu, 1989, p. 15)

Meanings, beliefs, and practices are produced through social relations, and their interaction within social fields is the central idea in the practice theory (Bourdieu, 1984 [1979], 1986). This view is also supported by researchers like Barker (2012, 2013) and Watson (2011), whose work has been discussed in Chaps. 2 and 3.

In the context of the present study, social constructionism suggests that researching HYP's social reality entails at least two levels of construction: how HYP make sense of their lives and how I, as a researcher, make sense of HYP's narratives and explicate them. By operating within significant social structural constraints, HYP can make sense of the reasons behind their homelessness, their street-based practices, and also their sexual choices, decisions, and practices. These descriptions are then filtered through how I make sense of them using the practice theory.

Research Strategy

One major challenge in designing research is to figure out ways to answer questions about a given social problem, the logic that helps produce new knowledge. Research strategies are such logics that provide a way to address the questions of *what* and *why* associated with a social problem (Blaikie, 2007). Generally, inductive and deductive reasoning have commonly been adopted in scientific enquiries. Inductive reasoning begins with data collection, which leads to a rigorous analysis of the data gathered and finally the production of discoveries (Bryman, 2012). Deductive reasoning is the reverse of induction, as it starts with a hypothetical statement, which leads to data collection, analysis, and finally, the confirmation or rejection of the given hypothesis, which has implications for the revision of a particular theory (Bryman, 2012).

Blaikie (2007) has criticised the linear reasoning evident in both the inductive and deductive approaches and proposed alternatives such as abductive reasoning, which

> incorporates what inductive and deductive research strategies ignore – the meanings and interpretations, the motives and intentions that people have in their everyday lives and which direct their behavior – and elevates them to the central place in social theory and research. (Blaikie, 2007, p. 90)

In line with philosophical assumptions, the present study is guided by the abductive research strategy. This is based on constructionist tradition and refers to the process of producing social scientific accounts using concepts and meanings individuals associate with their everyday activities (Blaikie, 2007). Constructionism holds that 'the social world is the world perceived and experienced by individuals from the "inside"' (Blaikie, 1993, p. 176). Therefore, social researchers' responsibility is to explore this insider view. The present study aims to locate social processes shaping HYP's life chances, notably their sexual experiences, which can be achieved through an exploration of how HYP make sense of their social and financial conditions, their social position within the broader society, and sex as a practice to secure needed resources.

Research Design and Methods

In consonance with the philosophical assumptions and abductive research strategy adopted, I used qualitative methods to explore HYP's lived experiences. Specifically, qualitative methods are well suited to understand contextual and social structural conditions within which individuals operate (Tracy, 2013).

Study Setting

The Islamic Republic of Pakistan is one of the world's most populous countries and is home to almost 208 million people (Pakistan Bureau of Statistics, 2017). The country appeared on the world's map in 1947 at the end of British rule in the Indian sub-continent, following a long struggle by Muslims to have a separate country to freely practise Islam. The geographic area of Pakistan spans a land mass of 796,096 km^2 and is divided into four provinces including Punjab, Sindh, Baluchistan, and Khyber Pakhtunkhwa, along with the Islamabad Capital Territory and Azad Jammu and Kashmir (PDHS, 2018).

The study was conducted in Rawalpindi, which is situated in Punjab, the largest province by population in Pakistan (PDHS, 2018). One major impetus to select Rawalpindi as the study setting was its significance as one of the major urban centres of Pakistan where a considerable number of HYP reside. While no official statistics are available regarding the estimated number of HYP, Emmanuel et al. (2005) estimate that a total of 3000–5000 'street children' reside in Rawalpindi. Other pragmatic reasons to select Rawalpindi as a study site were my previous experience of conducting research with homeless families and existing connections with some community-based organisations (CBOs) in the city.

Eligibility Criteria

Any social scientific enquiry into a given social problem must define the population groups under investigation (Caton, 1990). In this study, young people aged 16–25 years old who did not have a permanent dwelling were eligible to participate. The eligibility criteria were also guided by the recent social research into homelessness and youth studies. As far as the concept of homelessness is concerned, its definitions have varied considerably over decades. Nevertheless, one of the most discussed definitions is 'street homelessness', which Rossi et al. (1987) refer to as 'literal homelessness', which

> typically results from extreme poverty in housing markets with an inadequate supply of low-cost housing, especially for single persons…. The homeless are therefore best seen as the long-term very poor who cannot be taken care of by friends and family (or are rejected by them) and who have been unable, for a variety of reasons, to establish households of their own. (Rossi et al., 1987, p. 235)

Rossi et al. (1987) further distinguished the literal homeless from those who are 'precariously homed' (p. 235), people who experience unstable and insecure living conditions, such as those living with friends and relatives, leading to 'overcrowding and physically inadequate living settings' (Caton, 1990, p. 21). While these definitions capture distinct characteristics of individuals, a person having no permanent dwelling appears to be a common feature in classifying someone as homeless.

Youth refers to a phase of a person's life, which is understood and defined in various ways (Smith & Mills, 2019). A key variable used to define youth in most research is 'age'. In the work of social researchers like Beazley (2003), Tyler and Melander (2012), Barker (2012, 2013), and Watson (2011), the term 'young people' was used to refer to people aged between 15 and 25 years old. Guided by these sociological works, for the present research, the term 'homeless young people' refers to 16- to 25-year-olds who do not have permanent and secure accommodation.

Fieldwork

I moved from Australia to Pakistan to conduct the fieldwork from April to September 2016. I began the fieldwork by building rapport with staff from a local organisation working with HYP, who further assisted in recruiting HYP in the present study. The study used a purposive sampling technique, which is well-suited for studying a specific social phenomenon linked with a specific population group. Generally, in qualitative studies, a sample size of 30 participants is considered sufficient to achieve data saturation – a concept that refers to the quality and quantity of information collected in qualitative studies (Mason, 2010).

In the present study, data were gathered from a total of 29 HYP comprising nine cisgender heterosexual men and six women, seven cisgender gay men, and seven transgender heterosexual women. As the data collection went on, I listened to each interview's audio recording and noted the main themes that were raised. By the time I had conducted 29 interviews, I concluded that no new major themes were being raised, indicating that the data saturation had probably been achieved. At this point, I then proceeded to analyse the interviews in detail.

Interviews

In situations where it is not possible to meet research participants more than once, semi-structured interviews are recommended (Bernard, 2017). Therefore, semi-structured in-depth interviews were conducted with HYP in the Urdu language – a language that is widely used to communicate in Pakistan. However, a few interviews were conducted in Saraiki and Punjabi languages, as some HYP were not fluent in the Urdu language.

The interview guide consisted of four main sections: demographic information, reasons behind homelessness, experiences of street life, and sexual practices. Each interview began with an introduction and verbally informed consent followed by a casual conversation, generally about the weather, to create a relaxed environment. The first few questions were about HYP's demographic information in which I asked about their age, ethnic background, sexual/gender identity, and city of origin.

The second section explored HYP's pathways to homelessness. The third section explored HYP's street-based activities. Following this, questions related to sex were asked. This final set of questions led to a discussion around HYP's sexual partnerships, their beliefs about sex and HIV/STIs, and their sexual choices, decisions, and practices.

The first few interviews were closely analysed to determine shortcomings in phrasing, the sequence of questions, and the structure of the interview guide. As expected, the first few interviews revealed that HYP found it difficult to explicitly talk about sex. This issue was critical, as the major aim of the study was to explore HYP's sexual practices. This led me to rephrase some questions and restructure the interview guide in a way that all the questions related to sex were shifted to the end of the interview. Doing so was helpful because HYP generally felt more relaxed after talking about other things first. Moreover, I included a question related to whether it is difficult to talk about sex in Pakistan. This question helped HYP talk openly about the role of sex in their lives.

As soon as HYP began to talk about their sexual experiences, I paid closer attention to their responses and drew on various probing techniques to obtain rich information. I asked HYP open-ended questions and asked them to speak on a particular topic as much as they could and used the *silent probe* (Bernard, 2013, p. 187) such as nodding the head and using facial expressions to show HYP my interest in their stories. At times, to encourage HYP to continue to talk, I used the *echo probe* (Bernard, 2013, p. 187), repeating the last thing that HYP said.

In interviews conducted in the later stage of the fieldwork, I often used what Bernard (2013, p. 190) referred to as the *phased-assertion probe*, a technique by which researchers act like they already know about something to encourage HYP to open up. This probing technique was used specifically to obtain comparable narratives on a given topic. I often began by making a statement like 'some HYP told me that (for instance, some organisations educate on sexual health risks), are you also in contact with them?' This probing technique enabled HYP to talk more about their relationship with CBOs and how they had been helped or not.

Each interview was ended by asking HYP whether they wanted to ask me about anything else. After this, I thanked them for their participation in the research and presented them with 800 Pakistani rupees (AUD 10, as per the exchange rate when the fieldwork took place) as compensation for their time and travel-related expenses.

Data Analysis

Data analysis, in general, involves the exploration of ideas that help us explain various patterns (Bernard, 2013). I used a *thematic data analysis* technique to analyse information obtained from HYP. Thematic data analysis refers to systematically identifying and organising similarities and differences in the qualitative data, and it helps to offer insights into patterns of themes across a data set (Braun & Clarke, 2012). Specifically, I used this technique since it was sufficiently flexible to allow me to organise information in line with the theoretical concepts of capital, social fields, and habitus that guided this study, as well as identifying new or unexpected patterns in the data.

Figuring out thematic similarities and differences of the patterns in the qualitative data can be considered a task in which the researcher co-produces the data to interpret such patterns. Using the abductive research strategy, I first explored how HYP gave meanings to their living conditions and social experiences. Indeed, the process of analysing the data began at the fieldwork stage; after fully transcribing the first four interviews, I attempted to identify themes by reading and rereading the transcripts. This process helped me to emphasise targeted questions in future interviews.

The coding process began with importing all the interview transcripts into NVivo (version 10) software. Each interview was then read, and patterns of data were assigned headings/nodes. The coding frame provided me with a basis to interlink and reorganise different concepts and enabled me to structure the findings of the research. I then sought to relate concepts in the coding frame to the concepts in Bourdieu's theory (Bourdieu, 1984 [1979], 1986).

Key Ethical Considerations

The present research was approved (with reference number: HC16261) by Human Research Ethics Committee (HREC) of the University of New South Wales (UNSW). Key ethical guidelines concerning voluntary participation, informed consent, compensation for time and expenses incurred, and maintaining participants' confidentiality were observed throughout the research process. I anticipated that some participants might experience psychological distress due to the nature of the topics I intended to discuss with them. Therefore, I arranged to make free psychological counselling available to participants if they experienced distress. The organisation that helped me to recruit the study participants agreed to offer professional counselling if needed. While discussing the study with potential participants, I informed them about this service and that they were entitled to access it if they needed it. However, no participant reported distress, nor did any of them request this counselling service.

Since it was expected that participants might have limited literacy, I obtained verbal rather than written consent. The consent form was read aloud to participants, and their consent was audio recorded. Here, participants were informed about the voluntary nature of participation, their right to withdraw, and compensation for their time. Direct consent was obtained from participants aged 16–17 years old, as it was anticipated that the participants might have no or limited contact with their parents or legal guardians. Importantly, individuals of this age range are considered to be 'informed minors' – capable of providing informed consent (Sanci et al., 2004).

As participants were asked about their private lives, including their sexual experiences, it was expected that some of them might feel uncomfortable. Therefore, participants were advised that if they felt distressed or uncomfortable, the interview would be stopped to have a break and the interview would continue only if they agreed to do so.

I adopted various methods to protect participants' identities and ensure the confidentiality of the information obtained. For instance, during the fieldwork, each audio-taped interview was transferred to my password-protected personal laptop, with copies kept on a secure USB device. In addition to providing an orientation on data confidentiality to the transcriber, I masked participants' names and information regarding their origin in each audio-taped interview. In all the quotes from interviews included in the book, I have replaced participants' names with pseudonyms so that their confidentiality is maintained.

A Note on Reflexivity: Am I an Insider or Outsider?

Researchers' stance and the extent of their position as an *insider* or *outsider* in the research field can affect the research process. I identify myself as both an insider and outsider as far as the present research setting is concerned. I was born and raised in Pakistan, a country where talking about sex, except within marriage, is considered immoral. Before commencing this research, I was aware of the sensitive nature of the topic, at least in the Pakistani context, which led me to think of ways to make the research feasible. Since I had been working with some local organisations focusing on sexual and reproductive health issues among socially disadvantaged people, I drew on these existing connections to help me in the recruitment of research participants. Importantly, due to social and cultural constraints, I also knew that women would not be willing to discuss their sexual experiences with a male stranger. This led me to seek assistance from a local female interviewer, who helped me in recruiting some homeless young women in the study.

I also felt like an insider when it came to the language used to conduct the interviews. I can speak *Urdu*, *Punjabi*, and *Saraiki*, the languages used to communicate with HYP. However, I felt much more of an outsider when HYP used particular terms to refer to certain things. For example, when a transgender participant used the phrase: *phir maine guru ko chaila ki chatai pakra di* when referring to the process of gaining membership in peer groups. This phrase can be translated as *I offered some money to the group leader to become his/her student*. When the first time I heard this phrase, I asked the participant to explain what it meant. The participant then described the whole process of gaining membership in peer groups: drawing on existing connections in the street-based peer groups, being introduced to group leaders, requesting the group leader to include him in the group, and, if accepted, giving some money to the group leader as a token of respect. I was completely unfamiliar with the process of gaining membership in peer groups and the language used to describe it, which meant that I had to learn a new form of language that was a unique component of HYP life on the streets.

Another example where I felt like more of an outsider was occasions when I sensed that HYP did not expect me to be knowledgeable of their lifestyle. At times they considered me a medium through which their voices could be heard on the national and international levels. Many HYP, therefore, wanted to educate me about their lives. This happened most often during interviews with HYP with gender and sexually diverse identities. Often, before or during the interviews, these HYP asked about my sexual identity. They often assumed that a researcher who identifies himself as a cisgender heterosexual man may not be knowledgeable regarding social issues that people with diverse identities face in Pakistan. Therefore, HYP voluntarily described many issues they encountered in family life as well as after leaving home. For instance, many transgender participants talked about their childhood experiences. They told how behaving like women negatively affected their reputation within and outside their families and not being able to secure jobs in the formal economy contributed to their engagement in sex work. This rich information obtained from them contributed to my understanding that homelessness has many facets and there is a need to address these issues through continued research and advocacy.

Conclusion

In this chapter, I described the philosophical foundations that underpin the study methods that I used to conduct it. Based on the assumption that social reality is socially constructed, the study was underpinned by idealist ontology and constructionist epistemology. In consonance with the philosophical starting points, an abductive research strategy was adopted, which focused on the concepts and meanings HYP derived from their everyday activities.

In line with my ontological and epistemological stance, I adopted a qualitative method to undertake the study. I used semi-structured interviews as a way to obtain the qualitative data, which is analysed through a thematic analysis method. I also described how my position being an 'insider' as well as an 'outsider' may have influenced the conduct of the study.

The results produced by the use of the aforementioned methodology are presented in Chaps. 6, 7, and 8.

References

Baehr, P. (1990). Critical realism, cautionary realism. *The Sociological Review, 38*(4), 765–777.
Barker, J. D. (2012). Social capital, homeless young people and the family. *Journal of Youth Studies, 15*(6), 730–743.
Barker, J. D. (2013). Negative cultural capital and homeless young people. *Journal of Youth Studies, 16*(3), 358–374.

Beazley, H. (2003). Voices from the margins: Street children's subcultures in Indonesia. *Children's Geographies, 1*(2), 181–200.

Bernard, H. R. (2013). *Social research methods: Qualitative and quantitative approaches*. SAGE Publications.

Bernard, R. (2017). *Research methods in anthropology: Qualitative and quantitative approaches*. Rowman & Littlefield Publishers; Sixth edition (November 17, 2017).

Blaikie, N. (1993). *Approaches to social enquiry*. Polity Press.

Blaikie, N. (2007). *Approaches to social enquiry: Advancing knowledge*. Polity Press.

Bourdieu, P. (1984 [1979]). *Distinction: A social critique of the judgment of taste*. Harvard University Press.

Bourdieu, P. (1986). The forms of capital. In J. G. Richardson (Ed.), *Handbook of theory and research for the sociology* (pp. 241–258). Greenwood.

Bourdieu, P. (1989). Social space and symbolic power. *Sociological Theory, 7*(1), 14–25.

Braun, V., & Clarke, V. (2012). Thematic analysis. In H. Cooper, P. M. Camic, D. L. Long, A. T. Panter, D. Rindskopf, & K. J. Sher (Eds.), *APA handbooks in psychology®. APA handbook of research methods in psychology, Vol. 2. Research designs: Quantitative, qualitative, neuropsychological, and biological* (pp. 57–71). American Psychological Association.

Bryman, A. (2012). *Social research methods*. Oxford University Press.

Caton, C. L. (1990). *Homeless in America*. Oxford University Press.

Crotty, M. (1998). *The foundations of social research: Meaning and perspective in the research process*. SAGE Publications.

Emmanuel, F., Iqbal, F., & Khan, N. (2005). *Street children in Pakistan: A group at risk of HIV/ AIDS*. Retrieved from Pakistan.

Hirst, P. (2011). *Durkheim, Bernard and epistemology*. Routledge.

Mason, M. (2010). Sample size and saturation in PhD studies using qualitative interviews. *Forum: Qualitative Social Research, 11*(3), Art. 8.

Pakistan Bureau of Statistics. (2017). *Population census: Block wise provisional summary results of 6th population & housing census-2017* [As on January 03, 2018]. Retrieved from https:// www.pbs.gov.pk/content/block-wise-provisional-summary-results-6th-population-housing-census-2017-january-03-2018

PDHS. (2018). *Pakistan demographic and health survey – Key indicators report*. Retrieved from Islamabad.

Rossi, P. H., Wright, J. D., Fisher, G. A., & Willis, G. (1987). The urban homeless: Estimating composition and size. *Science, 235*(4794), 1336–1341.

Sanci, L. A., Swayer, S. M., Weller, P. J., Bond, L. M., & Patton, G. C. (2004). Youth health research ethics: Time for mature minor clause? *The Medical Journal of Australia, 180*(7), 336–338.

Smith, D. P., & Mills, S. (2019). The 'youth-fullness' of youth geographies: 'coming of age'? *Children's Geographies, 17*(1), 1–8.

Tracy, S. J. (2013). *Qualitative research methods: Collecting evidence, crafting analysis, communication impact*. Wiley-Blackwell.

Tyler, A. K., & Melander, A. L. (2012). Poor parenting and antisocial behaviour among homeless young adults: Links to dating violence perpetration and victimization. *Journal of Interpersonal Violence, 27*(7), 1357–1373.

Watson, J. (2011). Understanding survival sex: Young women, homelessness and intimate relationships. *Journal of Youth Studies, 14*(6), 639–655.

Chapter 6
Capital Deficit and Youth Homelessness

Family is the archetypal cradle of social capital and is the main site of accumulation and transmission of other forms of capital. Not being able to provide its members with adequate financial, cultural, and/or social resources means that a family may not be able to function as a source of social capital. This is because one of the key values of any form of capital is its capacity to be converted to other valued forms of capital. This chapter explores the conditions that lead to the decline of the family as a source of social capital, and how young people looked for other options to sustain it, and how this contributed to them becoming homeless.

This chapter has four main sections. This first section describes how limited financial capital held by families and cultural capital that homeless young people (HYP) embodied combined to produce contexts in which HYP had little choice but to leave their childhood homes. It particularly highlights how, in many cases, family poverty led parents to expect that HYP should quit formal education. Also, since many HYP felt obliged to support their parents, they left family homes and moved to an urban setting to engage in paid work. The second section identifies how the dominant heteronormative social structure played out to erode familial ties, which not only resulted in diminished financial, social, and emotional support but also contributed to violence against HYP who were gender or sexually diverse, forcing them to look for other forms of social support outside of their family homes. The third section describes how domestic violence rooted in certain familial and patriarchal values damaged the norms of trust and reciprocity within families. HYP who experienced domestic violence viewed their family lives as confinement rather than as a source of love, respect, and cooperation. The fourth section describes how, in one case, illicit drug use by a male participant disrupted familial relationships.

The chapter closes with a discussion of how the use of the concept of capital has helped to uncover social processes that contributed to HYP's homelessness through various pathways. Social structures like poverty, heteronormativity, patriarchy, and certain family norms played out to produce conditions in which families did not operate as sources of social capital. This impeded HYP's acquisition of cultural and

M. N. Noor, *Homeless Youth of Pakistan*, SpringerBriefs in Public Health, https://doi.org/10.1007/978-3-030-79305-0_6

other forms of capital, particularly access to educational and employment networks. In their effort to acquire social and financial capital, HYP drew on their informal networks on the streets, which, to some degree, provided them opportunities to survive and thrive. However, limited institutionalised cultural capital (Bourdieu, 1986), together with the stigma associated with diverse sexual/gender identities and illicit drug use, hindered HYP's access to the formal job market, indicating a process by which their social disadvantage was reproduced.

Poverty and Family Obligations

Most of the HYP came from families that did not have access to sufficient financial capital, and they believed this contributed to their homelessness. HYP tended to link it to their fathers' unemployment or insufficient income. Generally, in Pakistani rural society, gender roles are clearly defined: men are expected to work and provide financial support to their families while women are expected to remain at home, conduct household chores, and take care of children (Winkvist & Akhtar, 2000). This was also evident in the present study, as most of the HYP who came from rural areas mentioned that their mothers did not work outside the family home. HYP gave various reasons that contributed to their fathers' unemployment or insufficient income. For example, Zaheer described that since his father was his family's sole breadwinner, his income was insufficient to support a family of ten:

> It was necessary to leave home. My father is a fruit vendor, but he does not earn much. I am the oldest in my family and I have three younger brothers and six sisters. For this reason, I had to come here three years ago, I drive a rickshaw and can make five hundred rupees per day, and this is how I and my father run our home. (Zaheer,[1] Cisgender heterosexual man, 18)

Zaheer's account indicates that the family can act as a source of social capital under some conditions. In his case, the large family size meant that the financial capital held by Zaheer's family was too small to meet the everyday needs of each member. Since he was the first-born child, there were expectations attached to his position within the family. Being the oldest child, he was expected to try to generate income and reduce the financial hardship for his family. This finding is consistent with past research from Pakistan, which suggests that first-born children in families experiencing poverty are more likely to engage in paid work to help their families (Chaudhary & Khan, 2002; Qureshi et al., 2014).

Some HYP mentioned their fathers' inability to work due to sickness, physical disability, and old age. For example, Umair linked the disruption in his family income to his father's lower limb disability that made it difficult for him to walk.

---

[1] All names and other personal identifiers in this chapter have been changed to protect privacy and confidentiality.

The family's large family size and his brother's inability to work (due to illicit drug use) further exacerbated the family's financial hardship:

> I belong to a poor family. My father used to work as a tailor, but he does not work anymore due to his disability. My mother remains at home. I have two sisters and one elder brother who does not work due to his drug habit. Instead of supporting us, he expects us to support him. He does not come home for weeks. We could not even afford to rent a house. Therefore, I had to leave home and do something for my family. (Umair, Cisgender heterosexual man, 18)

Parveen and Qausar reported that their father could not work due to his illicit drug use, which they thought also negatively affected relationships within the family. Both women described that since their father was responsible for the financial hardship of their family, they did not want to interact with him anymore. Moreover, both sisters thought that their father had violated his obligations to the family, particularly by not providing them with financial support, and therefore it was justified to expel him from home. These women further reported that the inability of their father to work meant that they had to become the breadwinners for their family:

> I was a kid when my father started using powder [heroin]. We were living in a rented house. My mother was working as a housemaid. She used to go to neighbouring homes to do household chores for them such as washing clothes, dishwashing, and dusting, but we made her leave this work. She was sick. She had undergone surgery on her ovarian cyst. We said you take care of yourself; we will work. We never know this is going to happen to us; perhaps this was our destiny. (Qausar, Cisgender heterosexual woman, 16)

In Pakistan, domestic workers are usually women who provide services such as cleaning, washing, and childcare for affluent families. This work is usually based on an informal verbal contract, and they receive a marginal wage despite the physical work. Also, they risk being verbally, physically, and sexually abused by their employers (Malik et al., 2016). In this study, Qausar and Parveen believed that it was their moral responsibility to provide their mother with financial support so that their mother could avoid being exploited.

The view that if young people have no family, 'then self-evidently their family does not function as social capital' (Barker, 2012, p. 735) is supported by the present study. Mehwish described her homelessness as a result of the death of her husband and parents:

> I am the mother of one child, and I could not afford to raise him when my husband passed away three years ago. I could not go to my parents' home because both of my parents have also died. The circumstances were so hard. Living has become expensive. I rented a house and started working as a maid in a house in the neighbourhood. (Mehwish, Cisgender heterosexual woman, 25)

The death of her main caretakers including her husband and parents meant that she had few options she could draw on to support herself and her child. In her initial days of homelessness, she worked as a housemaid in a townhouse. There, she met another woman, also working as a housemaid. Mehwish further described how the abusive behaviour by her employer, and the low pay, led her to think about alternatives to generate income. Therefore, she discussed her concerns with the fellow housemaid who further connected her with a street-based group of sex workers. Since then, Mehwish was completely dependent on sex work, as she generated more income by doing this than she did by working as a housemaid.

The interviews also suggest that families typically could not facilitate HYP's accumulation of institutionalised cultural capital or, in other words, formal education. Coleman (1987) proposed something similar – the chances of children discontinuing education increase if families do not have sufficient financial resources (p. 381). Umair ended up leaving school because they wanted to engage in paid work to support their families:

> I used to study before I came here three years ago. I had to do it just because my family did not have money to support my education. (Umair, Cisgender heterosexual man, 18)

Nevertheless, most of these HYP felt obliged to help their parents who were experiencing financial hardship. This finding indicates that HYP gained some 'embodied cultural capital' (Bourdieu, 1986, p. 47) through their family histories and experiences, which also shaped their decision to look for other options of support outside the family home. In other words, HYP's sense of obligation to help parents represented their family values, embedded in the cultural blend of Islamic and South Asian heritage. Specifically, in Pakistani culture, parents' status is considered *second only to God*, and children are encouraged to be empathetic and obedient to their parents (Stewart et al., 2000, p. 336). Many HYP, therefore, described how they saw parents struggling to generate income, for which they felt a personal responsibility to help them out. It may also be worth noting that parents are expected/obliged to help their children, so if they violate this norm (through drug use, for example), the sense of responsibility to parents may be lifted/voided. Omar described how he felt obliged to help his family:

> It is not a big deal if you live for yourself. The great thing is that you live for others. I am doing all this because I love my family. (Omar, Cisgender gay man, 24)

The cultural capital that Omar embodied through his upbringing established his emotional connection to his family members. Indeed, he seemed proud about discontinuing education and leaving the family home, and this was driven by his intention to relieve his family's financial pressures. This is a clear example of what Warr (2005) calls 'horizontal or bonding' ties – the emotionally intense relationships based on social obligations to support family members. Therefore, the strong family norms evident in Omar's narrative meant that he never regretted discontinuing his education or leaving the family home; instead, he was proud of what he was doing for his family.

It is also important to note that many HYP described that they would not have left home if they had secured paid work in their native regions. Barker (2012) also suggests that although poverty is one of the major contributors to homelessness for young people (in Western settings at least), strong family norms can keep families together. As noted earlier, many HYP also described strong family norms and emotional connectedness. However, what led to their journey on the streets was fewer opportunities available in the rural areas where they lived. Zaheer compared work opportunities available in rural and urban settings:

> I came here to do some work because there is no promising work [opportunity] in my village. There are a few options available there, but you cannot make a good amount of money from them. Here, I drive a rickshaw and make money; this work is not available there. (Zaheer, Cisgender heterosexual man, 19)

HYP's narratives suggested how poverty, the job market of rural areas, and cultural norms of family life combined to produce a unique configuration of capital in HYP's families (i.e. limited financial capital, but for some, rich embodied cultural capital), which compelled them to look for other options of support outside their homes. Therefore, HYP mobilised their informal ties with extended family members, peers, and friends, who, to some extent, helped them to acquire social and financial capital that helped them to meet their personal and family needs. For example, Parveen described how she approached a friend who was already living on the streets to help her to engage in paid work:

> I asked my friend whether she can help me to find work. She then introduced me to these people because she was also doing this [sex work]. I knew her because she used to be my neighbour. (Parveen, Cisgender heterosexual woman, 18)

Since Parveen's father did not work due to his heroin use, she, being the oldest sibling at her family home, felt a responsibility to support her mother and younger siblings. She, therefore, sought support from her friend, who provided her with some 'bridging social capital' (Putnam, 1993), in that she connected Parveen to a group of street-based transgender people, who facilitated her sex work. Her narrative strongly supports the proposition that the accumulation and conversion of capital presupposes labour: some forms of social capital are built on the expenditure of time and attention (Bourdieu, 1986, p. 55). In Parveen's case, the elements of *closeness, trust,* and *cooperation* between herself and the friend evolve, which ultimately facilitated a productive action (Coleman, 1988; Putnam, 1993).

Overall, this section has identified how the interaction between financial, social, and cultural capital played out to shape HYP's decisions to leave home. The declining forms of capital (often in the family) precipitated a search for alternative sources, often drawing on extended family and friends (from bonding to bridging capital). This, in combination with embodied cultural capital – the social obligation to support parents – contributed to HYP's decision to leave home in search of paid work.

The Transgression of the Social Norms of Sexuality

Many HYP were transgender or gay and told stories of family rejection of these identities. For many of them, leaving home was seen to be a better option than living in restricted, unsupportive, or violent family environments. These family settings and relationships are set within the broader marginalisation of transgender and gay people in Pakistan.

Pakistan is governed by a combination of secular and Islamic laws according to which same-sex sex is illegal under section 377, *Unnatural Offenses* (Pakistan Penal Code (Act XLV of 1860)), 'an injunction that is inherited by British colonial rulers'

(Khan, 2014, p. 47). Under this law, a person who practises homosexual sex is punishable by heavy fines, prison, or even death. Although this law has rarely been invoked, its existence contributes significantly to the marginalisation of gender and sexually diverse communities (Khan, 2014).

In Pakistan, the dominant 'heteronormative social structure' that privileges heterosexuality sets up the social rejection and discrimination experienced by same-sex attracted men, women, and transgender people (Henshaw, 2014, p. 961). A principal contributor to the reinforcement of heteronormativity is the traditional religious values of Pakistani society, as in Islam homosexuality is considered immoral and therefore same-sex relations are criminalised (Alizai et al., 2017, p. 1216). HYP recognised this:

> We live in the Islamic Republic of Pakistan and Islam prohibits men to have sex with men.
> (Omar, Cisgender gay man, 24)

When asked what happens when a man comes out as gay, HYP reported that it could have very serious social consequences. Specifically, they believed that coming out as a gay man may negatively affect their relationships with family, relatives, and friends, resulting in discrimination and the fear of violence at work. Therefore, most of the gay men concealed their sexual orientation from their families and left homes for other reasons. Because the biological, patriarchal family is regarded as the central institution in Pakistani society, for individuals, the meaning of family is rooted in loyalty to its values, protecting its honour, taking care of other members, and procreation (Khan, 1997). Like many other HYP, Hassan also believed that 'coming out as a gay man would certainly result in the dishonour of his family in society' (Hassan, Cisgender heterosexual man, 24), and his family members (particularly his father) would not tolerate this. This finding strongly supports Bourdieu's (1986) proposition that social networks have institutionalised forms of *delegation*.

Bourdieu gives the example of how the head of the family is mandated to make decisions to preserve the totality of the family's social capital: financial, cultural, and social resources. This institutionalised delegation may also be authorised to expel 'embarrassing individuals' (p. 55) to save the social prestige of a given social group. This scenario was evident in the present study, particularly when Vaqas's family stopped supporting him after his sexual orientation was discovered, although he did not choose to disclose it. Vaqas described how he had intended to keep his sexuality secret, but his father read text messages he had exchanged with his partner. To prevent him from establishing sexual relationships with men, his parents forbid him to leave the family home. For Vaqas, his decision to leave home was better than living in a restricted and potentially violent environment:

> My father had suspicions that I am [sexually] attracted towards men, and he didn't like it at all. He used to keep an eye on me. He knew that I had sexual relationships with other men. He once read the text messages that I exchanged with my friend; it was a sex-related conversation. He then started monitoring my activities, like, where am I going, who am I meeting. My father and older brothers used to beat me up. They restricted me from going outside the home. I then decided to run away without letting them know. (Vaqas, Cisgender gay man, 17)

The interviews suggest that coming out as a gay man not only can lead to the loss of family but also impedes access to bridging social capital (Putnam, 1993). For instance, Emad would not even consider disclosing his sexual orientation to his straight friends as he feared they would stop talking to him:

> Straight people do not like gay men. They might think to end their friendship with me because I am a gay man. They believe being a gay man is a wrong thing. Therefore, I always pretend to be a straight man to avoid being ridiculed when I am with them. (Emad, Cisgender gay man, 25)

Emad identified himself as a gay man who was staying away from his family home so that he could be openly gay. He reported that because he was from conservative family background, coming out as gay man could be highly problematic and even dangerous for him. Although he did not want to talk more about his family, he said, 'they could go to every extent to save their honour'. By this, Emad was pointing to *honour killing*, a practice prevalent in the rural conservative society of Pakistan in which family members of a man, woman, or a transgender person kill them in response to their sex outside marriage or same-sex sex and the perceived shame this has brought on the family (Hussain, 2016, p. 70).

The stories of HYP who were transgender women also show how their families did not function as a source of social capital. Most of these HYP described that in their family homes, they experienced verbal and physical abuse by their male family members. For example, Talat was beaten up by her brothers due to her trans identity:

> I had been beaten up by my brothers several times because I talked like a woman. (Talat, Heterosexual transwoman, 24)

Although Talat's brothers did not accept her because she talked and acted like a woman, she was accepted by her mother and this was significant in Talat's life:

> Mother's love is unconditional, she asks me to come back, spend time at home, and enjoy the family life. (Talat, Heterosexual transwoman, 24)

This finding is consistent with the past research from Pakistan showing that women may be more accepting of family members with nonconforming gender identities (Alizai et al., 2017; Tabassum & Jamil, 2014). Nevertheless, due to predominant patriarchal values in Pakistani society, it is usually the case that families are headed by male family members, and this was the case for most HYP in this study. HYP reported that their fathers and older brothers acted in ways that protected their families' honour and prestige. Verbal and physical abuse by fathers and brothers was used to prevent HYP from talking or acting as gender nonconforming, such as wearing women's clothes, makeup, and jewellery. This was intended to prevent disrespect to their families. Talat described that to safeguard the family's honour, her brothers kept her inside the home and demanded that she talk and act like a man:

> My family members used to ridicule me, like; you are a *shemale*. This was all I used to hear from them, and it hurts. The way I walk, the way I talk, and my overall behaviour reflect a woman inside me, and this is natural. That is not my fault. This is how *Allah* [God] has created me. They ask me to remain at home, not to go outside because my relatives also used

to call me a shemale. My older brothers eventually said they do not accept the way I am, and they just kicked me out of the home. (Talat, Heterosexual transwoman, 24)

Talat's inclusion in her family became conditional: she was expected to play a traditional male role if she wanted to live at home. This finding is another clear example of how delegation functions to preserve the totality of social capital. In a society that is profoundly dominated by patriarchal and heteronormative values, for Talat, not being able to play a traditional male role made her ineligible to become a *custodian* (Bourdieu, 1986, p. 52) of the family's social capital. From a Bourdieusian perspective, each member of a given social group is required to be a custodian of norms, values, and the material resources connected to it, a precondition to sustain its existence (Bourdieu, 1986). Talat fell short of this criterion, as her trans identity meant that there was a disjuncture between how she identified herself and how she was expected to act in society. This contradiction led her family to stop supporting her for the 'embarrassment' she caused by acting like a woman, something that led to her expulsion from the family home. Although Talat remained connected with her mother after being expelled from home, her older brothers did not like it. Therefore, Talat would secretly talk to her mother via a mobile phone when her brothers were not around.

Importantly, the deterioration of HYP's familial relationships led them to seek alternative ways to gain social and financial capital. For instance, before leaving or being expelled from family homes, HYP accumulated some bridging social capital (Putnam, 1993), as they established connections outside the home, notably with gay and/or transgender communities, which helped them to gain membership in peer groups. These communities also acted as a gateway to a broad range of resources, which HYP accumulated and deployed to navigate their lives on the streets. HYP described how they gained physical protection, social, emotional, and financial support through peers as their alternative source of social capital. For example, Talat goes on to describe how she established connections with a transgender community through a transgender friend:

I joined a group through a friend from my native village. She is also a *moorat* [transgender woman]. For the initial few days, she managed my stay at a hotel. The United Hotel, near Pindi Chowk. She kept me there for two to three days. In those days, she made me meet some other transgender women who kept me afterwards. (Talat, Heterosexual transwoman, 24)

Talat's narrative indicates how her friend provided her with bridging social capital (Putnam, 1993) in that she connected her with people who might have different ethnic origins. One thing that united them all was their gender identity and experiences of discrimination in society, providing them with the impetus to expand their social network and help each other. Here, in addition to bridging social capital, Talat actively mobilised her erotic capital (Hakim, 2010, p. 500) to successfully navigate within sex working and dancing culture. Also, Talat's decision to undergo gender reassignment surgery was based on her wish to live like a woman, even being aware of the stigma attached to trans identity in Pakistan. Moreover, due to her personal experiences and by looking at the overall societal treatment of transgender people, Talat seemed certain that opportunities for her to live a *normal* life in society would not come. Therefore, Talat thought she was destined to dancing and sex work, and to do this successfully, she mobilised her erotic capital. However, drawing on her bridging social capital – the street-based peers – she acquired some cultural capital – the skills of beautification, dance, and sex work – and she enhanced her erotic capital, which she then converted into financial capital to meet her personal needs. It is important to note that HYP reported performing dance shows at wedding events, a legitimised cultural aspect of Pakistani society. Notably, when HYP mentioned dance work, they referred to mujra dance: a sexually suggestive dance that is generally attributed to transgender people and often to female dancers. Often, using sexually explicit songs, mujra dancers engage in explicit and sexually suggestive dancing to please their audience, who are generally men (Batool, 2015).

This section has analysed how the transgression of social norms of sexuality impacts the capacity of the family to act as a source of social capital for HYP. There was evidence of how heteronormativity played out in the disruption of HYP's familial relationships. Families stopped providing them social capital, as being a gay man or having trans identity was believed to be damaging families' honour in society, characterised by dominant heteronormative and patriarchal values.

Domestic Violence

Some HYP spoke about how their family lives were characterised by a lack of trust and cooperation. Their interviews suggest how physical abuse rooted in certain familial and patriarchal values deteriorated 'trust', which is an important condition for a family to function as social capital (Putnam, 1993). It appeared that instead of providing adequate social support, some HYP's families turned into what Wacquant (1998) calls an instrument of *surveillance* and *suspicion* (p. 25), as a few HYP reported that there were certain restrictions placed upon them by their families, and they would face physical abuse if they went against these restrictions. For example, Rashida described that her parents did not want her to spend time with friends, particularly at night. Generally, in Pakistan, parents decide the extent of young people's engagement with the world outside of the home, with whom they can socialise, where can they go, and for how long can they remain outside the home (Chattoo et al., 2004). Rashida discussed how her selection of friends and spending time with them was a contentious issue that she believed contributed to the physical abuse she experienced by her family:

> There were a few problems in my family life. My brothers used to scold me whenever I met friends. They thought my friends are bad people and they were particularly concerned when I came back home late at nights. I remember they had beaten me up very badly twice. I was fed up with all this and then I decided to leave home. (Rashida, Transgender heterosexual woman, 22)

Rashida came from a conservative rural family background where young people were expected to not spend excessive time with friends, particularly at night. She described that these family rules were intended to prevent young people from engaging in activities such as having sex before marriage, which is regarded as immoral:

> They [family members] were concerned about the things which happen outside the home like meeting bad friends or getting involved in sex. (Rashida, Transgender heterosexual woman, 22)

One woman, Saira, linked her homelessness to the physical abuse she experienced from her husband. She reported that her husband coerced her into sex work, which she was not willing to do. Before getting married she was not aware that sex work was her husband's family business. She described that she was physically abused several times by her husband because she did not want to engage in sex work:

> My husband always forced me to do [sex work]. I never thought of doing it. I was so young when I got married. I was the mother of two children, a boy and a girl, when my husband put me into this work. He was so cruel to me. I could not take good care of my children due to this and as a result, both of my children used to remain sick. I was beaten up whenever I resisted. I even got operated on for my neck injury which happened during one of our fights. I have been divorced recently but I can't go to my parents' home because they do not like me any more due to what I had been doing in the past. (Saira, Cisgender heterosexual woman, 25)

Saira initially resisted engaging in sex work but the physical abuse she experienced meant, ultimately, she relented. Her husband sent her to Dubai, where his sister was already doing sex work, while both of her children were in Pakistan. During her stay in Dubai, her son passed away and she was not sure about the reason that contributed to his death. This was the turning point in her life; after the tragic death of her son, she quit sex work, came back to Pakistan, sued and divorced her husband, and got legal custody of her daughter. However, by that time, her parents knew that she had been practising sex work, and this negatively affected her relationship with them, as sex work is perceived as shameful in conservative Pakistani society (Batool, 2015). She moved and sought help from her transgender cousin who introduced her to a 'new world' of the transgender community and dance shows. Since then, she lived with a small group of transgender people and young women to engage in dance work for her livelihood. However, dance work is also considered immoral and the people who are involved in this work are regarded as social outcasts (Pande, 2004). Therefore, to prevent her daughter from a stigmatising environment, she asked her mother to take care of her. However, Saira remains in contact with her daughter and provides financial support by sending money every month to her mother. Although Saira is not accepted by most of her family members, she has at least been helped by her mother in bringing up her daughter.

This section has identified how HYP's families turned into a source of *negative social capital* because they verbally and physically abused HYP due to their non-compliance with certain familial, heteronormative, and patriarchal norms. Because 'normal' family life is organised around the norms of trust, reciprocity, and obligations, violating these norms has prompted HYP to look for other options, setting their trajectories into the street life.

Illicit Drug Use

Farhan talked about how the use of illicit drugs, notably cannabis and heroin, disrupted their familial relationships, further leading to his homelessness. Specifically, illicit drug use not only contributed to his inability to work but also produced a context of distrust by family members. Farhan spoke about how his brothers stopped providing him with financial support as a way to stop him from buying drugs:

> I had conflicts with my brothers over my drug use. It was my brother's home, so he did not like me to stay there. He asked me to go and live on my own. My brother kicked me out with humiliation. I never harmed them, but they still think I am a bad person I don't know why? They become angry if I go home. They think I am there to ask for money and [they think] I [would] steal something away from them. (Farhan, Cisgender heterosexual man, 23)

Farhan was experiencing *literal homelessness* when his interview took place (Rossi et al., 1987, p. 235). He did not have access to any dwelling and, therefore, he would sleep in a public park since his older brothers expelled him from the family home. He initially used drugs for recreational purposes but, with time, he developed an addiction. As he was the youngest in his family and all his siblings were married, he recognised that if he had been able to stop using drugs, he might not have become homeless if his father was alive and was supporting him. Past research also suggests that people may cease their drug use and remain socially involved if they receive sufficient social and emotional support from close social networks, notably their families (Boyd & Mieczkowski, 1990; Sullivan et al., 2004; William & Latkin, 2007). Farhan's older brothers could not support him due to their parental responsibilities. He seldom went back to his home to see his mother because he was not welcomed by his brothers, who did not trust him due to his heroin use. While he was still in contact with his mother, who wanted him to return home, she could not help him as she was not the key decision-maker in the family. Therefore, Farhan remained on the street and supported himself by washing cars, scavenging, and begging. A large proportion of the money he earned was spent on buying drugs.

Conclusion

In this chapter, I have attempted to understand HYP's pathways to homelessness through Bourdieu's concepts of capital (Bourdieu, 1986). Generally, for a family to operate as a source of social capital, it must have access to financial and social resources and adhere to norms of social cohesion, trust, and reciprocity (Bourdieu, 1986; Coleman, 1988; Putnam, 1993). A family may not be able to provide social capital to its members if these elements are missing from it (Barker, 2012, p. 732). This view was supported by the results discussed above in this chapter. The decline of the family as a source of social capital, as described by HYP, was often the result of structural conditions like poverty, the constrained job market of rural areas, heteronormativity, patriarchy, and violation of the norms of trust and reciprocity. Together, these conditions produced a context in which families could not provide HYP with opportunities to thrive, contributing to their homelessness.

The analysis indicates a complex interplay between financial, social, and cultural capital in producing as well as reproducing HYP's social disadvantage. For example, limited financial capital meant that families were not able to provide formal education opportunities to HYP, which further hindered their access to the formal job market.

The analysis also illuminates a positive side of the family as a source of social capital. The strong family norms inculcated in HYP's embodied cultural capital (Bourdieu, 1986) gave them a sense of connectedness and belonging between them and their families, despite the experiences of financial hardship. Barker (2012), in his research from Australia, found something similar – despite leaving the family homes, young people had a connection to their families, even those who abused them. This connection, according to Barker (2012), often led to suffering, resentment, and pain. What stands out in the present study is HYP's *empathy* and *obedience* to their parents, rooted in Pakistani cultural heritage. The present study highlights HYP's moral responsiveness towards their parents' difficult financial circumstances. HYP's narratives indicate how they felt proud by leaving homes, engaging in paid work, meeting their families' subsistence needs, and supporting younger siblings' education- and marriage-related expenses, given that the elements of love, affection, emotional connectedness, and warmth existed between them and the families.

In many cases, the family did not operate as a form of social capital at all, particularly in the contexts where HYP transgressed social norms of sexuality or did not comply with strict family rules. Here, social structures, notably heteronormativity and patriarchy, acted to produce experiences of verbal and physical abuse, resulting in families' inability to function as a source of social capital, which further shaped HYP's perception that leaving home could be a better decision than living in a strict and abusive environment.

The decline of the family as a source of social capital meant that HYP were deprived of the social and financial support that families normally provide. Therefore, to accumulate this capital, HYP drew on their informal ties with extended family members, friends, and peers, another source of social capital, which they converted into financial and cultural capital. For instance, all of the HYP mentioned how their existing relationships on the streets helped them to secure paid work, although it was not well paid. In most cases, this was because their limited institutionalised cultural capital positioned them in a poor place in the formal job market. Therefore, most HYP converted their street-based social capital into cultural and erotic capital (Bourdieu, 1986; Hakim, 2010) – the acquisition of skills related to rickshaw driving, beautification, dancing, and sex work – that helped HYP to meet their personal and family needs.

References

Alizai, A., Doneys, P., & Doane, D. L. (2017). Impact of gender binarism on Hijras' life course and their access to fundamental human rights in Pakistan. *Journal of Homosexuality, 64*(9), 1214–1240.

Barker, J. D. (2012). Social capital, homeless young people and the family. *Journal of Youth Studies, 15*(6), 730–743.

Batool, S. F. (2015). *New media, masculinity and mujra dance in Pakistan.* Centre of Media and Film Studies, SOAS, University of London.

Bourdieu, P. (1986). The forms of capital. In J. G. Richardson (Ed.), *Handbook of theory and research for the sociology* (pp. 241–258). Greenwood.

Boyd, C. J., & Mieczkowski, T. (1990). Drug use, health, family and social support in "crack" cocaine users. *Addictive Behaviors, 15*(5), 481–485.

Chattoo, S., Atkin, K., & McNeish, D. (2004). *Young people of Pakistani origin and their families: Implications for providing support to young people and their families.* Retrieved from https://www.dmss.co.uk/pdfs/young-people-of-pakistani-origin-and-their-families-final-report.pdf

Chaudhary, M. A., & Khan, F. H. (2002). Economic and social determinants of child labor: A case study of Dera Ismail Khan, Pakistan. *The Lahore Journal of Economics, 7*(2), 15–40.

Coleman, J. (1987). The creation and destruction of social capital: Implications for the law. *Notre Dame Journal of Law, Ethics & Public Policy, 3*, 375.

Coleman, J. S. (1988). Social capital in the creation of human capital. *The American Journal of Sociology, 94*, S95–S120.

Hakim, C. (2010). Erotic capital. *European Sociological Review, 26*(5), 499–518.

Henshaw, A. L. (2014). Geographies of tolerance: Human development, heteronormativity, and religion. *Sexuality & Culture, 18*(4), 959–976.

Hussain, M. S. (2016). History, law and vernacular knowledge: The threat to women's collective representation under the guise of androgyny in Pakistan. *King's Student Law Review, 7*, 64.

Khan, B. (1997). Not-so-gay life in Pakistan. In *Islamic homosexualities: Culture, history, and literature* (pp. 275–296). New York University Press.

Khan, F. A. (2014). *Khwaja Sira: Culture, identity politics, and "transgender" activism in Pakistan.* Syracuse University.

Malik, A. A., Majid, H., & Fateh, H. (2016). *Women in Pakistan's urban informal economy: Vulnerabilities, opportunities and policy solutions.* Washington: Urban Institute and Oxfam. Retrieved from https://www.urban.org/research/publication/women-pakistans-urban-informal-economy/view/full_report

Pakistan Penal Code (Act XLV of 1860). Retrieved from http://www.pakistani.org/pakistan/legislation/1860/actXLVof1860.html

Pande, R. (2004). The politics of dance in Pakistan. *International Feminist Journal of Politics, 6*(3), 508–514.

Putnam, R. D. (1993). The prosperous community. *The American Prospect, 4*(13), 35–42.

Qureshi, M. G., Nazir, S., & Hina, H. (2014). *Child work and schooling in Pakistan-to what extent poverty and other demographic and parental background matter?* Retrieved from Islamabad.

Rossi, P. H., Wright, J. D., Fisher, G. A., & Willis, G. (1987). The urban homeless: Estimating composition and size. *Science, 235*(4794), 1336–1341.

Stewart, S. M., Bond, M. H., Ho, L., Zaman, R. M., Dar, R., & Anwar, M. (2000). Perceptions of parents and adolescent outcomes in Pakistan. *British Journal of Developmental Psychology, 18*(3), 335–352.

Sullivan, T. N., Kung, E. M., & Farrell, A. D. (2004). Relationship between witnessing violence and drug use initiation among rural adolescents: Parental monitoring and family support as protective factors. *Journal of Clinical Child & Adolescent Psychology, 33*(3), 488–498.

Tabassum, S., & Jamil, S. (2014). Plight of marginalization: Educational issues of transgender community in Pakistan. *Review of Arts and Humanities, 3*(1), 107–122.

Wacquant, L. J. (1998). Negative social capital: State breakdown and social destitution in America's urban core. *Netherlands Journal of Housing and the Built Environment, 13*(1), 25.

Warr, D. J. (2005). Social networks in a 'discredited' neighbourhood. *Journal of Sociology, 41*(3), 285–308.

William, C. T., & Latkin, C. A. (2007). Neighborhood socioeconomic status, personal network attributes, and use of heroin and cocaine. *American Journal of Preventive Medicine, 32*(6 Suppl), S203–S210.

Winkvist, A., & Akhtar, H. Z. (2000). God should give daughters to rich families only: Attitudes towards childbearing among low-income women in Punjab, Pakistan. *Social Science & Medicine, 51*(1), 73–81.

Chapter 7
The Street Field: A Capital-Building Site

Because the family lives of homeless young people (HYP) were characterised by the *capital deficit* (Green, 2008, p. 39), they looked for other options of support outside the family home. This chapter describes how HYP entered a street-based social space where they acquired various forms of capital essential to their survival on the streets.

The chapter is composed of two main sections. The first section analyses how using bridging social capital (Putnam, 1993) – the existing social ties on the streets – HYP entered a social space, something like 'the street field' (Shammas & Sandberg, 2015, p. 196). The field had its internal *logic of practice*, which Bourdieu (1990, p. 80) calls doxa, which gave HYP a sense of their position within the field and the broader social world, and also made them aware of the internal social dynamics of the field. The second section describes how the street field helped HYP in many ways to accumulate financial capital that enabled HYP to meet their personal and, in some cases, their family needs. Since, in many peer groups, financial gains were contingent on dancing and sex work, HYP needed to accumulate some 'embodied' and 'objectified/material' cultural capital to enhance their 'erotic portfolio', the most sought out element by the male clients of sex work and *sexually suggestive dancing*. In other words, HYP learned skills related to beautification, dancing, mannerisms, communication styles, and other sexual skills, all of which make up the erotic capital (Hakim, 2010, p. 500), which they further mobilised in dancing and sex work to generate financial capital. Furthermore, material resources like makeup items, clothes, rented rooms, mobile phones and, in one case, a motorbike helped HYP to successfully practise dancing and sex work.

The chapter closes with a discussion of how the concepts of capital, street field, and doxa (Bourdieu, 1986, 1989, 1990, 1998) helped to identify HYP's agential ways by which they attempted to mitigate their circumstances of marginalisation. Notably, the results show how various forms of capital played out in shaping HYP's street-based practices. To enter the street field, HYP deployed social capital – existing connections on the streets. The field then helped HYP to learn new skills (i.e.

M. N. Noor, *Homeless Youth of Pakistan*, SpringerBriefs in Public Health, https://doi.org/10.1007/978-3-030-79305-0_7

dancing, communication, beautification, and sex working skills) and use material resources so that they could generate incomes through dancing and sex work. However, the field had its internal logic of practice – members who did not comply with the rules and norms were expelled by group leaders, as they were perceived to be a threat to the existence of the group. Although dancing and sex work were believed to be the most viable options to generate incomes, enough to meet HYP's everyday needs, this work may be perceived as socially undesirable or unacceptable by the general public and may serve to reinforce HYP's marginalisation.

The Street Field

HYP established connections with peers who lived on the streets before leaving family homes. These connections acted as a source of social capital in that they helped HYP to enter the street field – an activity-specific social space of hierarchical relationships occupied by young people who share somewhat similar experiences of poverty, family abuse, societal discrimination, and homelessness, and which promotes the norms of cooperation to facilitate each other's access to social and financial capital, essential to survive in homelessness.

It appeared that HYP gained membership in three types of peer groups: groups based on sexual/gender identities, groups based on ethnic origin, and groups organised around hotel-based sex work networks. While these groups varied concerning their composition and functioning, across them there were some common features: each had membership rules; there was shared recognition about who was the group's leader; and there were shared norms of trust and reciprocity and rules to regulate members' conduct.

An important precondition to enter the street field was HYP's acquaintance with any of its existing members, something that established 'trust' between HYP and other group members, without which entry into the field would be denied. Here, HYP's connections on the streets with relatives and peers played a pivotal role to help them out: they acted as a source of bridging social capital (Putnam, 1993) in that they initially provided HYP with things like accommodation and food and, to some extent, helped them to engage in paid work and then connected them with peer groups. For instance, Laila described how, after leaving home, a friend accommodated her, and this further helped her to gain membership in an organised peer group:

> I had a good friend of mine who was living [there]. I was constantly in contact with her. She would always say that I would always be welcomed if I wanted to go to her. I stayed at her place for an initial couple of days during which I made more friends and started living with them (Laila,[1] Transgender heterosexual woman, 22).

---

[1] All names and other personal identifiers in this chapter have been changed to protect privacy and confidentiality.

Many HYP mentioned how their friends helped them to find paid work. Omar, for example, described how he left home in search of paid work, which he secured with the help of a friend:

> I was aware that my friend was living near the Temple Road and was working as a house-painter and could earn two to three hundred rupees per day by doing that work. I straight away went to him and started doing the same. This is how I started my life [here] (Omar, Cisgender gay man, 23).

In addition to providing help regarding accommodation and engagement in paid work, peers guided HYP on how gaining membership in peer groups could optimise their chances of securing protection against verbal/physical abuse by the general public and optimise other income generation opportunities. Hassan, a gay man, described how, in his initial days of homelessness, his peers advised him to join a group based on diverse sexual/gender identities if he wanted to be safe on the streets:

> I was told by some friends from the start that if I wanted to be safe, I would need to join a group. It's just like how a politician needs to choose a political party and the party supports him. Similarly, I had to choose a group of *shemales*,[2] led by a guru [leader]. She [the leader] promised me to ensure my safety and said no one could dare to touch me if I joined them (Hassan, Cisgender gay man, 23).

When talking about the *group of* shemales, Hassan was referring to something like the *house/ball community* in the United States that provides social support to gay men and transgender people of colour who experience social marginalisation (Phillips et al., 2011, p. 516). Similar to the house/ball community, the group that Hassan joined was organised in a way that entailed hierarchical *relationships of exchange* (Bourdieu, 1998, p. 26). The group was led by an experienced transgender woman leader, called 'guru'. Hassan joined this group because he feared violence from his ex-partner. Hassan said because his ex-partner worried that Hassan would disclose his same-sex sexual orientation to people around them, he harassed Hassan so that he would move away. Therefore, Hassan looked for a community that could not only embrace his sexual identity but also protect him, and this is where one of his friends who was connected with a transgender community advised him to join them for protection.

Nevertheless, the street field operated following its doxa (Bourdieu, 1990, p. 67) – the taken-for-granted and unquestioned norms regarding young people's membership and their conduct within the field. These norms involved recognising the authority of a group leader, embracing the values of trust and reciprocity, and the possibility of expulsion from peer groups if a member engaged in misconduct. The doxa regulated the behaviour of group members so that the existence of the street field could be sustained and the capital available within it continued to be available.

Those who strictly followed the norms of the street field were permitted to access a range of valuable resources attached to it, which HYP further mobilised around dancing and sex work and generated income. For instance, to practise sexually suggestive dancing successfully, HYP needed to increase what Hakim (2010) calls

---

[2] A slang commonly used to refer to transgender people in Pakistan.

erotic capital – something necessary to please their audience. This analysis strongly supports Bourdieu's (1986) proposition that the interconvertibility of capital types shape social practice. Here, HYP used social capital (peers) to obtain cultural capital (skills of beautification), something that used to increase their erotic capital (attractiveness) that further helped them to generate financial capital (money). When it came to sex work, many HYP spoke about how peers taught them various ways to interact with potential clients on the streets: standing on the roadsides, making eye contact, and winking at potential clients and having sex with them – the processes that eventually helped HYP to earn some money.

Rules for Membership

One of the basic prerequisites to enter the street field was to recognise the authority of group leaders, who were typically the most senior and experienced persons. Since peer groups varied in their composition and functioning, the characteristics of group leaders also varied. For example, while groups based on diverse sexual/gender identities were usually led by the most experienced transgender women, other groups were led by cisgender men. Transgender women leaders usually acted like 'mothers', as they provided the junior group members with social and emotional support and mentoring. However, the leaders of hotel-based sex working networks were generally cisgender men, as their masculinity gave them a status that enabled them to negotiate with the police about the illegal sex work businesses they were running.

In addition to recognising the authority of group leaders, HYP needed to deploy certain forms of capital to gain acceptance in the street field. For instance, Hassan deployed a combination of social, financial, cultural, and erotic capital to gain membership in a peer group formed based on diverse sexual/gender identities and where financial gains were contingent on dancing and sex work:

> I was introduced to my group through other people from my community [sexual minorities]. You get to know each other in everyday casual meetups, for example in public parks and then they hook you up with other people. This is how we enter groups…. There are rules that we need to follow to gain membership in a group. As a starting point, you need to meet a guru [transgender leader] and offer her some money. It's like paying an admission fee to enter a university and then it becomes the university's responsibility to educate you. The guru-chela relationship is just like a relationship between a teacher and a student or a mother and a child. Once you have established this relationship, you will be cared for and you don't have to worry about anything. The amount of money you give to a guru depends on how much she demands, but some gurus may leave it to you; how much you can afford to pay (Hassan, Cisgender gay man, 23).

The above narrative indicates that Hassan recognised the importance of gaining membership in the street field, as it provided him opportunities to enter a safe social milieu and to 'survive in the face of adversity' (Barker, 2013, p. 370). However, to achieve these benefits, he deployed his bridging social capital (Putnam, 1993) in that he was introduced to his group leader through his peers. Also, giving some money to the group leader as a token of respect points to his mobilisation of financial and cultural (i.e. values of respect toward a group leader) capital (Bourdieu, 1986). His interview also provides evidence of how erotic capital – being a young man who can provide sexual services to male clients – also helped him to secure membership in the group and how this erotic capital was most valued among peers:

> Being able to secure more clients can have a tremendous impact on your reputation within the group. Everyone appreciates and acknowledges that you are a highly demanded person, you are into the business, and you are earning money, very nice, etc. (Hassan, Cisgender gay man, 23).

Sohail's interview also suggests how his erotic capital (Hakim, 2010) enabled him to enter a hotel-based sex working network. He was referring to his youth and attractive looks – the *natural immutable attributes* (Green, 2008, p. 29) of erotic capital – as a criterion based on which he was suggested by his peers to enter the sex working network. Notably, these physical characteristics, Sohail told, were usually sought after by male clients. According to Berti (2003), typically, male sex workers who provide sexual services to male clients in small-scale hotels in Pakistan can be as young as 13 years old. Although Sohail did not like practising sex work, he did it to survive. He spoke about how during the initial days of his homelessness, he used to scavenge and sell discarded items to scrap dealers until his friend, who was affiliated with a hotel, asked Sohail to join him:

> There was a guy with who I had a friendship here. He used to hawk for a hotel. I would meet him and borrow cigarettes at the hotel and at that time I couldn't even afford a single cigarette. I came to know about him later when I witnessed him negotiating on the money with a client. He also tempted me to do the same because he knew I was a suitable person for this work. I then also started doing it because I needed money (Sohail, Cisgender heterosexual man, 16).

Sohail talked about the composition of the group he joined. He said that the sex work business was collectively run by a hotel owner, an accountant, some hawkers, male sex workers, and the police in a hotel. Each of these people had specific roles to play. The hotel owner was the head, the accountant handled cash, the hawkers marketed for hotel rooms by shouting on the roadsides, and other young men provided sexual services to male clients. According to Sohail, the police took money from the accountant regularly so that they would not harass the hawkers and sex workers. The money received from a client was divided into five equal parts, Sohail, the owner, the hawker, the sex worker, and the policemen. Because Sohail was younger than 18 years of age, he was not eligible to open a bank account where he could deposit the money he earned. He kept his money with a nearby retail shopkeeper who charged a fee to keep his money safe.

Sohail appeared to have mixed feelings of *satisfaction* and *regret* about his sex work. For example, he seemed satisfied with the amount of money he generated from sex work. In other words, the financial capital he was generating from sex work was sufficient to meet his personal and family needs, which might not be possible if he continued to perform scavenging. On the other hand, he regretted practising sex work, as he believed that he was committing a 'wrongdoing' and if his family knew it, they would kill him. Several times in his interview, he referred back to his family poverty by saying that

> If I had money, I would have been doing some business. I would not be into this wrongdoing, but I am helpless, I have no other choice (Sohail, Cisgender heterosexual man, 16).

However, Sohail did not think of quitting sex work because he was earning a good amount of money from it. Also, as per his verbal contract with the hotel owner, he would not be able to re-enter the network if he quit practising sex work because many young men were in a similar untenable situation as Sohail was and could be easily convinced to join. That is, Sohail was easily replaceable. This finding strongly supports Bourdieu's (1998) proposition that there are limits to how the game can be played within a given social field, and these limits are set by its doxa. For Sohail, despite having negative feelings regarding his sex work, he did not want to leave his group because he knew that leaving the group would ultimately result in losing income that was important to support his family experiencing financial hardship.

A few interviews suggest the extent to which *ethnic capital* – social ties within an identifiable ethnic community (Zhou & Lin, 2005, p. 261) – was most valued to secure membership in some peer groups. For example, Bilal, who identified himself as a Saraiki[3] by ethnicity, gained membership in a group based on Saraiki young men from his native area. He said that to gain membership in this group, a person was required to be from the same native region and be acquainted with some of its members. In addition to having a specific ethnic identity, recognising the authority of the group appeared to be another important precondition to gain membership in Bilal's group. Notably, in Bilal's group, financial gains were contingent on manual work, and his leader always made decisions about the group mobility; the group would move between various cities in search of better wages:

> I am living with six other men who are all from my village. We all were in Karachi before moving here because he [the leader] said [here], there might be more work opportunities (Bilal, Cisgender heterosexual man, 17).

Bilal also talked about how his leader directed the group members not to mix with local people, as it might carry the risk of violence and financial loss. He further gave a few examples of how his peers were robbed and beaten by some local men. Most of the members in Bilal's group were masseurs who carried oil bottles on a tray and went to public parks to give massages to men. Bilal described that one of his peers was robbed by his clients, who took him to a quiet street and snatched his money and a mobile phone. This finding also points to the dark side of social capital – social connectedness may not be always invariably positive, it may sometimes bring negative outcome (Field, 2008). Perhaps, Bilal's leader was concerned about the 'norms of trust', an essential element that transforms social connectedness into meaningful and facilitative ties (Putnam, 1993), something that was missing in Bilal's relationship with the locals.

---

[3] An ethnic majority in South Punjab province of Pakistan.

   This section highlighted various rules what Bourdieu (1998) refers to as doxa that determined whether someone was eligible to enter the street field. HYP wanted to enter a social milieu that could ensure their physical safety and social support, as well as providing them work opportunities to better manage their homelessness. To participate in this field, they deployed certain forms of capital: social, financial, cultural, erotic, and ethnic (Bourdieu, 1986; Hakim, 2010; Zhou & Lin, 2005). Specifically, existing ties on the streets provided them with bridging social capital to connect them with peer groups (Putnam, 1993). HYP mobilised cultural, financial, and erotic capital when it came to gaining membership in peer groups led by transgender leaders and/or where financial gains were contingent on dancing and sex work. Additionally, a few HYP deployed their ethnic capital to secure membership in peer groups based on ethnic identities. However, one common feature across all these peer groups was that they were led by group leaders and HYP needed to recognise the leaders' authority to gain membership in the street field.

Norms of Reciprocity

For HYP to maintain their membership in peer groups, it was necessary to follow the norms of *trust* and *reciprocity* (Putnam, 1993). Indeed, these norms were in place to strengthen ties between group members so that they could be protected. Hassan used a metaphor to describe how peer groups ensure physical protection:

> Individually, we all are weak, but group life can protect us. It's just like one plus one equals eleven (Hassan, Cisgender gay man, 23).

   To receive this level of protection, group members were encouraged to care for each other. Therefore, HYP helped each other cook food, share accommodation- and food-related expenses, provide financial support and help peers in securing paid work, and give emotional support to each other. Additionally, group leaders also managed group members' living expenses; they paid for grocery items and accommodation and divided all the expenses they incurred among everyone in the groups at the end of each month. HYP's narratives implied that these norms of sharing and reciprocity were important not only to reduce group members' financial burden but also in terms of strengthening the ties between them. Specifically, Bilal indicated how peer groups provided some social capital to make things easier for each other:

> We all live like brothers. We equally divide the expenses related to grocery and we cook food together and I think it is very useful because we don't have to buy ready-made food from outside. It makes food less expensive. The good thing is that if someone is not working and don't have money, others can feed him and they don't even say they are giving you a favour (Bilal, Cisgender heterosexual man, 17).

   Many HYP talked about how peers, to some degree, were obliged to provide financial support to those who needed it. Particularly, this norm mostly benefitted those who had not been able to secure paid work and were obliged to provide financial support to their families. One woman, Jaweria, reported that peers helped each other to meet their family needs:

Living together is beneficial because at least friends know if someone is in trouble. For example, if someone is running out of money, others can help by making her meet their clients. If this does not solve the problem and someone needs money for her family, friends can send money to them and then the problem is solved (Jaweria, Cisgender heterosexual woman, 23).

Jaweria's group comprised both men and women, whereby men were responsible for securing accommodation and bringing clients, while women practised sex work. In her group, the men took money from clients and gave part of the earnings to the women. Although the men and women lived together as per a verbal business agreement, they also helped each other if someone experienced trouble. This ensured that their business was not affected.

Some HYP talked about the emotional support they received from peer groups. For instance, Talat described how she often felt distressed by recalling her experiences of violence and expulsion from home by her older brothers and how her friends acted as a source of happiness for her:

I do not live with my family anymore. For me, my friends are my family members now. We help each other through our ups and downs. We also fight just like siblings do in a family, but we remain happy together (Talat, Heterosexual transwoman, 24).

Talat recognised that 'cooperation' (Coleman, 1988) between friends was not to be taken for granted but had to be continuously worked on through an environment of mutual respect. She believed that because all her peers were living away from their families, it was important for them to care for each other; otherwise it would be difficult to survive homelessness.

Norms of Punishment

Many HYP reported that practices like stealing, misbehaviour with peers, and disloyalty to group leaders were not tolerated, and a person found to be involved in these acts was considered a threat to the existence of peer groups. Accordingly, such persons were subject to punishment or expulsion. Hassan described how group members could lose social capital if they broke the group code of conduct:

Persons who do something wrong must be punished by the guru [the group leader]. For example, the group leader can stop providing things like food, clothes, makeup, or even clients, if you have stolen something or fought with your group member and you are the culprit. The group leader can even ask all to boycott such persons for some days if somebody tries to talk to them, s/he would also be subject to punishment (Hassan, Cisgender gay man, 23).

Hassan further told that if something had been stolen from his group and the culprit was not known, the group leader would financially punish the entire group. The group leader would divide the estimated cost of that stolen item and attribute it to everyone in the group and collect money to buy a new one. He described how others could pay the price for someone else's wrongdoing:

It also happens that you never did something wrong, but you must pay the price. If some-one's makeup kit has been stolen and people start to blame each other, the group leader can, for example, take five hundred rupees from each person and buy a new one (Hassan, Cisgender gay man, 23).

The proposition that in given social field individuals are connected through rela-tionships of *material and/or symbolic exchanges* (Bourdieu, 1986, p. 51) is strongly supported by HYP's narratives. For example, group leaders' provision of social support to junior members was an *investment* (p. 48), in which they were entitled to *credit* (p. 51) in the form of recognition, respect, and, sometimes, financial capital. Jaweria described that if group members received clients through group leaders and did not reveal the exact amount of money they earned or did not give her group leader his/her share, they were considered 'disloyal' and would be immediately expelled from the group:

I must give half of the money I earn if I attended a client through him. If I don't do this, I wouldn't be able to work with them. He can straight away kick me out (Jaweria, Cisgender heterosexual woman, 23).

Nevertheless, hiding money from group leaders was believed to be very difficult and rare. Vaqas described that his group, based on diverse sexual/gender identities, was close-knit and so if a person cheated, they could not hide from their peers:

You must have to give your group leader her share at any cost. Suppose if I cheat on her, she will instruct her subordinates to follow me, and they cannot ignore her advice. The group leader knows we people have a limited social circle. She will certainly find me out someday and take her share (Vaqas, Cisgender gay man, 17).

Also, the street field appeared to be an important 'capital-building setting' (Bryant, 2018, p. 986). As noted earlier, in most peer groups, financial gains were contingent on dancing and sex work, and for HYP to practise these works success-fully, they needed to acquire adequate skills. Here, the street field provided HYP opportunities to obtain these forms of resources: cultural capital in embodied and objectified/material state (Bourdieu, 1986, pp. 47-50), relevant to dancing and sex work, practised to generate some financial capital. When asked what skills HYP acquired to perform dancing, most of the HYP emphasised beautification and sev-eral ways that made them look sexually suggestive while entertaining their audience.

Conclusion

In this chapter, I used the concepts of capital, social fields, and doxa (Bourdieu, 1986, 1990, 1998) to uncover social mechanisms through which HYP navigated their lives in homelessness. Since HYP's lives were characterised by the capital deficit, they looked for other options of support outside their family homes. Here, existing relationships on the streets provided HYP with bridging social capital (Putnam, 1993), particularly in connecting them to peer groups, which further gave

them access to social and cultural capital. Using these capital types, HYP then accumulated the financial capital needed to better navigate their homelessness.

However, gaining membership in peer groups was not a straightforward process.
It was like entering the street field (Shammas & Sandberg, 2015, p. 196) – an
activity-specific social space of 'hierarchical relationships' occupied by young people who shared somewhat similar experiences in that their lives were characterised
by capital deficit, something that contributed to their homelessness. Also, the street
field promoted the norms of *mutual cooperation* (Coleman, 1988) to facilitate each
other's access to essential forms of capital, notably social and financial capital.

The street field contained individuals who were *dominant* as well as those who
were *dominated* (Bourdieu, 1998, p. 40). These positions were defined based on the
extent to which individuals possessed a specific *volume* and *composition* of social,
cultural, and financial capital (Bourdieu, 1986, p. 48). For instance, group leaders
were usually the most senior and experienced members in peer groups, indicating
their *symbolic efficacy* of cultural capital (Bourdieu, 1986, p. 49), and this is what
enabled them to dominate the junior or less experienced group members.

Specifically, this domination of group leaders was legitimised by the 'doxa – of
the game' (Bourdieu, 1990, p. 66), played within the street field: the taken-for-
granted shared norms and understandings guiding HYP about how to act within the
field, also specifying what was considered as *good* or *bad* conduct. The doxa established the conditions upon which HYP's involvement and membership in the street
field were structured. For instance, HYP were advised to meet group leaders,
express their interest to them, and, if accepted as members, they were required to
give group leaders money or gifts as a token of respect. In other words, the doxa
meant that HYP were required to deploy a range of resources or capitals, specific to
the nature and composition of peer groups. Entry into the peer groups, based on
sexual/gender diverse identities and hotel-based sex working networks, presup-
posed the deployment of social, erotic, and, to some extent, financial capital. For
instance, HYP needed to mobilise their existing ties on the streets, their sexual/
gender identities, interest in performing dance and/or sex work, and some money to
be given as a token of respect to a group leader to enter peer groups formed along
with the basis of sexual/gender identities. Besides, a few HYP deployed their ethnic
capital to gain memberships in peer groups based on ethnic origins.

The doxa promoted norms of sharing, trust, and reciprocity to ensure the mutual
benefits of members as well as to sustain the existence of the field. Therefore, members found to be involved in stealing, misbehaviour, and cheating on group leaders
were financially punished or expelled to control social behaviour within the field,
without which the street 'field would become anarchic and cease function'
(Thomson, 2008, p. 68), something that could be a threat to its existence.

The street field also determined how HYP would be positioned within broader
society. For example, the financial gains in the field were contingent on dancing and
sex work, the taboo works, usually attributed to the professions of social outcasts in
Pakistan (Batool, 2015). However, within the field, the members supported each
other to practise these works, without being judgmental, as individuals could

generate more financial capital than by doing house painting, scavenging, or other labourer work.

The results discussed in this chapter indicate the extent to which HYP displayed agency within significant structural constraints. They improvised with limited resources available on the streets, and most of the HYP strategically chose dancing and sex work as professions, as they knew that this kind of work could help them to generate incomes, sufficient to meet personal, and, in some cases, their family needs. Therefore, they participated in the street field and gained social capital – relations with peers – who helped them to accumulate financial capital, largely through dancing and sex work. Nevertheless, this kind of work had implications for the reinforcement of their social marginalisation due to the stigma associated with dance and sex work in Pakistan. People who practise it are considered social outcasts, and it can reduce or diminish social support from other important social circles, like the family.

References

Barker, J. D. (2013). Negative cultural capital and homeless young. *Journal of Youth Studies, 16*(3), 358–374.

Batool, S. F. (2015). New media, masculinity and mujra dance in Pakistan. In *Centre of Media and Film Studies*. SOAS, University of London.

Berti, S. (2003). *Rights of the child in Pakistan*. Retrieved from Geneva:

Bourdieu, P. (1986). The forms of capital. In J. G. Richardson (Ed.), *Handbook of theory and research for the sociology* (pp. 241–258). Greenwood.

Bourdieu, P. (1989). Social space and symbolic power. *Sociological Theory, 7*(1), 14–25.

Bourdieu, P. (1990). *The logic of practice*. (N. Richard, Trans.). Stanford University Press.

Bourdieu, P. (1998). *On television*. (P. P. Ferguson, Trans.). The New Press.

Bryant, J. (2018). Building inclusion, maintaining marginality: how social and health services act as capital for young substance users. *Journal of Youth Studies, 21*(7), 983–998.

Coleman, J. S. (1988). Social capital in the creation of human capital. *The American Journal of Sociology, 94*, S95–S120.

Field, J. (2008). *Social capital*. Routledge.

Green, A. I. (2008). The social organization of desire: The sexual fields approach. *Sociological Theory, 26*(1), 25.

Hakim, C. (2010). Erotic capital. *European Sociological Review, 26*(5), 499–518.

Phillips, G., Peterson, J., Binson, D., Hidalgo, J., Magnus, M., & Group, Y. o. c. S. I. S. (2011). House/ball culture and adolescent African-American transgender persons and men who have sex with men: a synthesis of the literature. *AIDS Care, 23*(4), 515–520.

Putnam, R. D. (1993). The prosperous community. *The American Prospect, 4*(13), 35–42.

Shammas, V. L., & Sandberg, S. (2015). Habitus, capital, and conflict: Bringing Bourdieusian field theory to criminology. *Criminology & Criminal Justice, 16*(2), 195–213.

Thomson, P. (2008). Field. In M. Grenfell (Ed.), *Pierre Bourdieu: Key concepts* (pp. 67–81). Acumen Publishing Limited.

Zhou, M., & Lin, M. (2005). Community transformation and the formation of ethnic capital: Immigrant Chinese communities in the United States. *Journal of Chinese Overseas, 1*(2), 260–284.

Chapter 8
Sexual Risk-Taking: Competing Priorities of Capital-Building, Physical Safety, and Sexual Health

The content of this chapter is based on a study[1] that I previously published in the journal *Health and Social Care in the Community* (Noor et al., 2020). Here, I expand my analysis through the concept of *habitus* – a system of dispositions formed through past and ongoing experiences that guides individuals to evaluate social situations and act accordingly. Because homeless young people (HYP), to survive, sought memberships in peer groups where income generation was largely dependent on sex work, this means that they were sexually active and had concurrent sexual partnerships, which could put them at risk of HIV and other sexually transmitted infections (STIs) (Gross & Tyring, 2011). This chapter, therefore, explores HYP's sexual partnerships, the resources accrued from them, their knowledge regarding sexual health risks, and their sexual choices, decisions, and practices. I explore these interrelated practices using the concepts of capital and habitus (Bourdieu, 1984 [1979], 1986), which help to uncover the logic underpinning sex and sexual risk-taking.

There are four sections to this chapter. The first section describes some of how HYP gained social and financial capital by engaging in concurrent sexual partnerships (Bourdieu, 1986). Specifically, long-term intimate partners acted as a source of horizontal social capital (Warr, 2005, p. 286) – emotionally intense relationships that also provide resources like physical protection and money. In addition, sex work helped HYP to generate incomes essential to meet their personal and, sometimes, family needs. Based on the view that individuals' sexual behaviour may be shaped by their knowledge regarding sexual health risks (Gillmore et al., 2002; Zhao et al., 2012), the second section describes the information that HYP possessed regarding the nature, transmission, prevention, and treatment of HIV/STIs. This section specifically highlights how some community-based organisations (CBOs) acted as a source

---

[1] This chapter draws on content from: Noor et al. (2020). "Sexual risk-taking among homeless young people in Pakistan", *Health and Social Care in the Community*. https://doi.org/10.1111/hsc.13220. © 2020 John Wiley & Sons Ltd. Used with permission.

© The Author(s), under exclusive license to Springer Nature Switzerland AG 2021
M. N. Noor, *Homeless Youth of Pakistan*, SpringerBriefs in Public Health, https://doi.org/10.1007/978-3-030-79305-0_8

of *formal social capital* (Wacquant, 1998, p. 28) in that they helped HYP to build *cultural health capital* (Shim, 2010, p. 2) – biomedical information regarding sexual health risks and safety. To explore whether HYP's sexual health knowledge contributed to consistent condom use, the third section explores their sexual practices and reasons behind particular sexual acts. It particularly highlights how HYP's habitus of instability (Barker, 2016, p. 671) – produced through their difficult and unstable past histories – created expectations that their futures would be insecure. Their sexual decision making was impacted by this habitus or set of expectations about the future. Notably, social obligations in intimate partnerships, financial considerations, and fear of violence from clients collectively produced a context in which protection from HIV/STIs became secondary to maintaining relationships, income generation, and physical safety. The fourth section explores whether they took any measures (other than condoms) to reduce their risk of HIV/STIs. This section describes alternative methods of risk reduction, such as oral sex, anal douching, and the use of specific sexual positions, that HYP believed would protect them from HIV/STIs.

The chapter closes with a discussion of how Bourdieu's concepts of capital and habitus helped to understand HYP's sexual risk-taking. Since HYP's lives were characterised by a capital deficit (Green, 2008), this condition shaped their habitus and the HYP's worldview that they were socially and financially vulnerable and that this situation would remain unchanged. HYP were aware of the importance of the social and financial capital they were accumulating on the street, without which their survival would be difficult. Social obligations in intimate partnerships, fear of violence by clients, and the desire to maximise incomes from sex work produced a context of competing priorities, where HYP neglected sexual health risks attached to condomless sex. While alternative strategies were used to protect against sexual health risks, these were not always effective and might inadvertently increase their risk of HIV/STIs.

Sex, Relationships, and Benefits

According to Pakistani law, people found to be engaging in sex outside marriage and homosexual sex are criminalised and can be subject to punishments including fines, prison, or even death (Toor, 2007). Although HYP were aware of these socio-sexual norms, they gave various reasons to engage in sex outside marriage and same-sex sex. Hassan, for instance, believed sex was necessary to fulfil his erotic appetite:

> I think sex is a natural physical need, just like food for a body. Everyone needs to have sex at some time, after a week or two. I also need it for my physical satisfaction (Hassan,[2] Cisgender gay man, 23).

---

[2] To ensure confidentiality, HYP's original names and geographical locations within Rawalpindi were masked by the use of pseudonyms.

Ghalib described how he believed that, for gay men living in Pakistan, establishing long-term intimate relationships with men was an alternative arrangement for marriage:

As far as I am concerned, it is not possible to get married to a woman. I cannot even think of doing it, but society, including family, cannot accept it. My parents don't even know what I do here. I lied to them that I work in a hotel. They must be concerned that now that I have grown up, I should get married, but I cannot do it. Here, I have a boyfriend I am happy with it. My parents often ask me to get married, but I haven't refused them straightaway. I told them that I will get married when I have a better job (Ghalib, Cisgender gay man, 25).

Ghalib was one of many HYP who did not disclose to his family that he was a gay man because he feared rejection by his parents. Heterosexual marriage is a crucial organiser in Pakistani society, as it is in many others, and Ghalib's parents would have been seeking marriage for him as a way to prevent him from having sex outside of marriage (which is seen as sinful and shameful) and so that the family could gain a daughter-in-law who could help with household chores (Buriro & Endut, 2016).

HYP described how, through intimate partnerships, they accrued some horizontal social capital as a means to gain affection, companionship, and emotional support from their intimate partners (Warr, 2005, p. 286). Parveen did not want to get married because, being the oldest child, she was obliged to support her mother and siblings, which she did through sex work. She knew that sex work was taboo in Pakistan and was aware it was unlikely that a man would marry her. However, to obtain intimacy, she had entered a relationship with a man, outside of wedlock:

I feel good when my boyfriend is around. He comes, we lay down in the bed, we become physical, and we do not necessarily have sex every time. That is not a 'sex' that I have with my clients. I cannot spend hours with them, I simply want them to do their work [sex] and leave because it's just my business (Parveen, Cisgender woman, 18).

In Pakistan, women are expected to preserve their virginity until they get married (Khan, 2011). Those who are unable to do so are considered unmarriageable or are likely to be divorced soon after marriage. Importantly, in the Pakistani context, marriage implies a relationship between families rather than two individuals. Generally, a marriage cannot take place without the consent and agreement of the couple's families (Hamid et al., 2011). As Parveen was engaged in sex work, and because her father was an illicit drug user, she would likely be considered, by herself and others, as unmarriageable. Therefore, to obtain intimacy, a sense of belonging to someone, and a feeling of being valued and loved, she entered an intimate partnership outside of marriage.

Another woman, Saira, reported how her intimate partner provided her with physical protection. Saira did dance work and she felt vulnerable to verbal, physical, and sexual abuse by men at dance events. Her intimate relationships secured physical protection, and her partner was influential financially, socially, and politically:

People know that I am a weak person. This is obvious that no respectable woman in our society would do dance work. Men had beaten me up a few times in the past and it gave me a sense of insecurity but thanks to the man who protects me. I am sure people will face serious consequences if they bully me now (Saira, Cisgender heterosexual woman, 25).

Saira also described a few incidents when men physically abused her in the past in response to her refusal to have sex with them:

Even though I had quit sex work, people often proposed me to have sex while performing on dance shows. I would tell them that I don't do this work anymore. A person once took me to a room and asked for sex. He tried to rape me when I resisted. I somehow hit him with my nails and in reaction to this, he started beating me up with a belt until I fainted. My friends then took me home and took care of me (Saira, Cisgender heterosexual woman, 25).

Most of the HYP reported engaging in sex work. Indeed, many had sought membership in peer groups where financial gains were contingent on sex work. Although a few HYP described having been engaged in jobs like street vending or house painting, they had left such jobs, as they had found that they could earn more money in sex work. Besides, some HYP mentioned that they were unsuccessful in securing jobs in the formal economy due to their low levels of education or that they were transgender or gay. Therefore, HYP believed that sex work was the most viable option to generate income, enough to meet their personal and, sometimes, family needs.

This section indicates that sexual practice helped HYP to accumulate social and financial capital. While sex outside marriage and sex between men were prohibited socially, religiously, and legally in the country, HYP engaged in such practices to fulfil their erotic appetites as well as to gain needed resources like physical protection, social and emotional support, and money. The next section explores HYP's knowledge regarding HIV/STIs and sexual safety. This analysis will further untangle how their knowledge shaped their choices, decisions, and practices concerning sex.

Knowledge of HIV/STIs

HYP had a mixture of good and patchy knowledge regarding sexual health risks and safety. Local CBOs appeared to be an important source of information about biomedical knowledge regarding HIV/STIs, something Shim (2010, p. 2) refers to as 'cultural health capital'. In this way, CBOs and their staff acted as a source of 'formal social capital' (Wacquant, 1998, p. 28) that could be drawn on by HYP to increase their safety during sex work. Many HYP like Talat recognised the importance of health promotion experts to gain information regarding HIV/STIs and condom use, which they did not have before meeting them:

I never knew about risks related to sex because most people in my community had no awareness regarding this, so they do not discuss it. I heard about HIV infection, hepatitis, and condom use from people from a non-governmental organisation (NGO) and it was quite worrisome because I had always been having sex without using condoms (Talat, Heterosexual transwoman, 24).

Because HYP received education from health promotion experts, they were able to distinguish between symptomatic and asymptomatic STIs. Indeed, HYP had access to free medical care from local sexual health organisations. When Ghalib experienced urethral discharge, he consulted an STI expert within a CBO, who identified it as a gonorrhoeal infection:

I once experienced the discharge of semen along with pus and blood. It was quite worrisome for me and I had to consult a doctor who diagnosed it as *sozak* [gonorrhoea] and treated it accordingly (Ghalib, Cisgender gay man, 25).

Similarly, some women talked about how they believed that excessive vaginal discharge might indicate leucorrhoea – a bacterial STI showing symptoms such as having a thick whitish or yellowish vaginal discharge accompanied by profuse foul odour (Abid et al., 2016). Jaweria also linked leucorrhoea with excessive vaginal discharge:

There is a lot of smelly [vaginal] discharge in the leucorrhoea which can also give a lot of headaches and it also sometimes causes rashes around the vaginal area (Jaweria, Cisgender woman, 23).

Almost all of the HYP were aware that STIs could also be asymptomatic. For instance, Parveen reported that because STIs could be asymptomatic, it was more likely that a person having sex with multiple partners could be at an increased risk of infection:

People who have sex with many partners carry pathogens. For clients who visit me, it is more likely that they visit other sex workers too. They may concurrently have had sex with hijras [transgender people], and other women and you do not know who is infected (Parveen, Cisgender heterosexual woman, 18).

However, many HYP, based on information derived from health promotion experts, believed that one could prevent HIV/STIs even when they had many partners if condoms were used consistently. Many HYP reported that they regularly received condoms from health promotion experts free of cost. Emad described how a gay friend who was working with a CBO often provided information relating to STIs and safer sex methods and gave him condoms:

I think using condoms is the best way to prevent diseases. We call it a penis cover. It acts as a shield against diseases. My gay friend who works for an organisation has told me about this. I also receive free condoms from him (Emad, Cisgender gay man, 25).

While many HYP were aware of the nature, transmission, and prevention regarding HIV/STIs, some of them held beliefs that did not align with biomedical knowledge of HIV/AIDS. For instance, some HYP believed that HIV infection could not be managed and, therefore, was a death sentence. Indeed, many of them were not able to differentiate HIV from AIDS. When asked why they believed so, these HYP reported how seeing their peers die from AIDS led them to believe that there was no medication to manage the infection. However, Hassan was aware that HIV is a chronic infection that could be managed through adherence to antiretroviral treatment (ART):

You cannot say HIV infection has no treatment. Although it remains with a person for his/her whole life, one can live a normal life by taking a pill every day. It's even safe to have sex without using condoms as far as the viral load is undetectable (Hassan, Cisgender gay man, 23).

Hassan's knowledge of HIV and ART was based on his personal experience of being a person living with HIV, something that he revealed during an informal conversation after his interview took place. Hassan described that he thought he would soon die when he tested seropositive. However, a clinician from an ART centre in Pakistan told him how by adhering to ART, he could live a healthy life. It is important to note that a total of 33 ART centres are operating in the country, where people living with HIV can receive ART free of cost. While Hassan believed that he was living a healthier life despite his HIV-positive status, he did not disclose his HIV status to his family members, peers, and clients, other than a few close friends, due to the social stigma associated with HIV in Pakistan. These findings imply that CBOs were mainly promoting safer sex and reducing HIV-related stigma was a secondary concern. This was perhaps the reason that almost all of the HYP, except Hassan, believed that HIV was a death sentence.

This analysis in this section demonstrates that HYP had a mixture of both good and patchy knowledge of sexual health risks. CBOs were a source of formal social capital (Wacquant, 1998, p. 28), helping HYP to build some cultural health capital (Shim, 2010, p. 2) – basic biomedical knowledge about HIV/STIs, their modes of transmission, prevention, and, to some extent, treatment. Therefore, many HYP could differentiate between symptomatic and asymptomatic STIs and knew the importance of consistent condom use, with one homeless young man viewing HIV as a chronic infection that could be managed by adhering to ART. As multiple studies reviewed in Chap. 3 suggest that having good knowledge regarding HIV/STIs may be insufficient to affect practice, and it is important to consider social structural forces when assessing individuals' sexual behaviour. Therefore, the next section explores HYP's sexual choices, decisions, and practices and analyses what contributed to decisions about sexual safety in sexual encounters with intimate partners and clients.

Sexual Risk-Taking

Despite having basic knowledge about sexual health risks and safety, most of the HYP engaged in condomless sex with intimate partners and clients. Their decision to engage in condomless sex appeared to be shaped by what Barker (2016, p. 671) calls the habitus of instability – a worldview of social and financial insecurity and instability formed through past experiences of familial disruption, societal discrimination, limited financial resources, and unstable living conditions. This worldview gave HYP a sense of their place in the world and enabled them to view themselves as having few resources and little capacity to change their circumstances. Therefore, HYP aimed to sustain social capital (Bourdieu, 1986) when it came to their sexual choices in intimate relationships because they believed that negotiating condoms with intimate partners would negatively affect 'trust' in these relationships. Saira described that she was not concerned about condoms, as she believed her partner was faithful to her:

> We do not use condoms because we do not need to. We are very close to each other. I trust that he does not have sex with anyone except me and he thinks the same about me (Saira, Cisgender heterosexual woman, 25).

Most of the HYP who practised sex work talked about how, to maximise their income, they often chose to practise condomless sex with clients and were offered more money to have condomless sex. Here, the maximisation of financial capital was preferred over sexual safety:

> I do not bother who I have sex with because sex work is the only way by which I can earn some money. I would not be able to feed myself if I don't do it. I never send my clients back because my only concern is money. Even if there is someone infected and can pay what I demand, I will happily accept it (Vaqas, Cisgender gay man, 17).

Although many HYP preferred using condoms, they could not use them, particularly when 'clients offer more money for not using them' (Emad, Cisgender gay man, 25). Additionally, they told stories of how they feared violence from clients who were intoxicated and were adamant that they did not want to use condoms:

> Drunk clients have a thing in their mind that they can have sex the way they want. Such clients then do not listen to me and I have no option left but to follow them (Talat, Heterosexual transwoman, 24).

Mehwish reported that some of her clients believed that condom use could reduce physical pleasure from sex and, therefore, they did not want to use condoms. To sustain a good relationship with clients who were her source of income, she often engaged in condomless sex. Since Mehwish's livelihood was completely dependent on sex work, she could not afford to lose her clients. Her financial hardship drove her decision to engage in condomless sex, despite her awareness of the risk of HIV infection:

> Some clients say they cannot enjoy sex by using a condom. They keep on insisting that they wanted to have sex without using condoms and I cannot then resist them (Mehwish, Cisgender heterosexual woman, 25).

Omar mentioned that he purposefully chose to avoid condoms because he believed that condom use might prolong sexual activity:

> I do not like my clients using condoms because I do not want them to last longer. I think the skin to skin contact during sexual intercourse heats a penis due to which a client can enjoy more and reach a climax earlier. Putting a condom on can prolong sexual activity which causes discomfort to me (Omar, Cisgender gay man, 24).

While Omar knew he was taking a risk by engaging in condomless sexual intercourse, he used strategies, notably, oral sex and anal douching, as substitutes for condom use, a theme that the chapter will turn to next.

The results of this section support the view that sexual behaviour may not necessarily be shaped by individuals' knowledge of sexual health risks and safety and that other structural and contextual factors shape sexual practices (Dunn et al., 2017; MacPhail & Campbell, 2001; Tadele, 2010). The results indicate that HYP's ongoing conditions of insecurity and instability shaped their habitus – the worldview that their social and financial insecurity would always prevail. Based on this worldview, HYP aimed to preserve forms of capital they accumulated on the streets for their survival. Social obligations in intimate relationships, the desire to maximise income, and power imbalances between HYP and clients produced a context of competing priorities in which sexual safety became a secondary concern. However, because HYP knew that condomless sex could expose them to sexual health risks, they used a variety of alternative strategies that they believed could reduce the risk of HIV/STIs, a description of which is given in the next section.

Sexual Health Risk Reduction Strategies

Peers helped HYP to develop a 'localised' cultural health capital – a *common sense* understanding of health and illness that HYP and their peers operated with (Warwick et al., 1988, p. 213). HYP spoke about how peers often advised them to use methods like withdrawal, masturbation, post-sex anal douching, oral sex, specific sexual positions, and refusing sex with people who looked a certain way to reduce the risk of HIV/STIs during condomless sex. These strategies were well-intentioned and grounded in everyday sexual experiences. However, if based on inaccurate knowledge of HIV/STI transmission risks or false optimism, this localised cultural health capital could inadvertently put HYP at higher risk.

A few HYP mentioned how they used the withdrawal method to reduce the risk of HIV/STIs during condomless sex with clients. Rashida, for instance, talked about how she negotiated withdrawal before ejaculation if her clients did not like to use condoms:

> The other method is not letting a client cum inside because some do not want to use condoms. I do not let such clients cum inside me. I always caution them that if you do not want to use condoms, make sure that withdraw before you cum. This is how they remain careful (Rashida, Transgender heterosexual woman, 22).

In contrast to Rashida's experience that clients would agree to withdraw before ejaculation, Omar reported that in his experience of sex work, clients never wanted to do so, as they believed it could reduce physical pleasure from sex; something that clients did not expect when paying for sex. Omar, based on a friend's advice, using the method of post-sex douching, believing it could reduce the risk of HIV/STIs:

> I have a friend from Lahore who taught me how to clean myself from inside after having sex without using a condom. I have a shower hose in my bathroom. Each time I have sex with a client, I go to the bathroom and wash my bottom with a high-pressure water stream and try to take semen out of my body. This is how I clean myself from inside (Omar, Cisgender gay man, 24).

While Omar believed that post-sex anal douching could protect him against STIs, from a biomedical perspective, anal/vaginal douching can lead to skin damage, which can potentially increase the chances of HIV transmission during condomless sex (Carballo-Dieguez et al., 2008). There is evidence that people who engage in post-sex anal/vaginal douching are at far greater risk of HIV (Millett et al., 2006, 2007; Wang et al., 2005). Omar's practice of anal douching was based on localised cultural health capital – beliefs about sexual safety acquired from peers – and while it was well-intentioned, it might have increased his risk of HIV/STIs.

Furthermore, Emad described using a specific position during sexual intercourse as a method to protect himself if his clients did not want to use condoms. It is important to note that Emad's concept of using a specific position during the sexual intercourse was substantially different from how *strategic positioning* is formally understood. Notably, strategic positioning, sometimes called seropositioning, is an HIV risk-reduction method used by serodiscordant couples in which an HIV-positive partner takes the receptive role during intercourse while the HIV-negative person takes the insertive role (Van De Ven et al., 2002). Research suggests that while strategic positioning does not eliminate the risk of HIV transmission, it does appear to reduce the risk of HIV transmission if practised consistently (Jin et al., 2010; Vittinghoff et al., 1999). Emad described that if his clients did not want to use condoms, he would be on top of his client while taking the receptive role, irrespective of the client's serostatus. While Emad knew that condomless sex was a risky practice, he practised it, particularly when a client offered him more money than usual. He further reported that peers often discussed their sexual experiences with clients with each other and suggested certain methods to prevent HIV, one of which was his version of positioning:

> In the case of condomless sex, I try to be on top of my client [while taking a receptive role]. It is safe to have sex in this way because I think semen does not travel deeper inside if you are on top (Emad, Cisgender gay man, 25).

A few HYP reported that as they had to attend to many clients daily, they tried not only to reduce the risk of HIV/STIs but also to minimise the time they spent having sex with each client. They believed oral sex and masturbation were two useful methods to achieve both goals. For instance, Hassan mentioned oral sex when asked if he used a different risk reduction method besides condom use:

> It has become a trend among young people that they want to cum in the mouth. They mostly ask me to have oral sex and if not, I try my best to have oral sex with clients and do not give them a chance to have [penetrative] sex and I think it is safe as well. Doing oral sex makes things easier. For example, you do not have to take baths again and again; you just wash your mouth and that's it (Hassan, Cisgender gay man, 23).

Naila also talked about how she practised oral sex or masturbated clients who she believed were unsafe partners:

> I do not usually have [penetrative] sex with people having rashes on their bodies. They may look fine but when they take their clothes off, I decide whether I should have sex or not. I

refuse them in a way that they do not feel bad. I just try to not let them penetrate in me. I either do oral sex or masturbate them but no anal (Naila, Heterosexual transwoman, 24).

For many HYP, sexual decision-making was primarily contingent on their assessment of clients' physical appearance. HYP reported abstaining from sex with people who looked dirty, skinny, or over 50 years old. Sohail mentioned how he believed that he became sick after having sex with a client who looked dirty:

I am now very careful in deciding who I should have sex with. I completely avoid those who look dirty. I simply reject them because they can make me sick. I remember how I once became sick by having sex with a dirty person. I had to go to a hospital and spend four thousand rupees [almost AUD 40] for the treatment of rashes I had on my whole body (Sohail, Cisgender heterosexual man, 16).

As described in preceding chapters, Sohail sold sex in collaboration with a local small-scale hotel that ensured the physical protection of street-based sex workers. Therefore, he did not fear rejecting clients whom he believed had STIs. When asked why he believed it was risky to have sex with people with a dirty physical appearance, he mentioned his personal experience of being sick. Similarly, a few HYP reported abstaining from having sex with persons who appeared skinny.

The results of this section illustrate that, since HYP were aware that they were at risk of HIV/STIs due to inconsistently using condoms with multiple partners, they actively looked for and used alternative risk-reduction methods, some of which might reduce risk, while others did not. Generally, drawing on peers' advice (a localised form of cultural health capital), they used methods like oral sex, masturbation, withdrawal, using specific sex positions, and post-sex anal douching and believed that these methods would reduce their risk of HIV/STIs.

Conclusion

This chapter has used the concepts of capital and habitus to understand HYP's logic of sexual risk-taking (Bourdieu, 1984 [1979], 1986). It provides original insights into the social conditions and contexts of competing priorities, where HYP's sexual safety became a secondary concern, despite being aware of sexual health risks associated with condomless sex. The results indicate that HYP's ongoing social and financial instability and uncertainty shaped their habitus of instability – a worldview that HYP were socially disadvantaged and that this disadvantage would be ongoing (Barker, 2016).

Most of the HYP obtained 'cultural health capital' (Shim, 2010, p. 2) – biomedical information regarding sexual health risks and safety – through their connections with CBOs. These organisations were a formal source of social capital (Wacquant, 1998, p. 28), as they not only educated HYP on sexual health risks but also provided them with free medical care and condoms. Most of the HYP could distinguish between symptomatic and asymptomatic STIs, their sexual transmission, prevention, and treatment. This knowledge, however, did not always help HYP when it came to making decisions regarding condom use in sexual encounters with intimate partners and clients. Simply put, there was a gap between what HYP learned from CBOs and what they practised. These findings do not support the view that HYP's sexual risk-taking was simply the result of insufficient knowledge regarding HIV/ STIs (Allahqoli et al., 2018; Busza et al., 2011; Sherman et al., 2005).

Since intimate partners provided HYP with physical protection, affection, and social, emotional, and financial support, they believed negotiating condom use with them would damage *trust* (Putnam, 1993) that could disrupt these intimate relationships. Similarly, in sex work, maximising income generation and avoiding violence by intoxicated clients took primacy over condom use. HYP could not risk losing these important sources of social capital in circumstances surrounded by familial disruption, discrimination, and marginalisation. The social and emotional support obtained from intimate partners outweighed HYP's concerns over sexual health risks.

HYP's past experiences suggested that negotiating condom use with clients could produce verbal or physical abuse or at least dissatisfaction from customers, and this produced expectations that condom use was not possible in many interactions with clients. Additionally, HYP knew that clients might not like condom use due to the belief that it reduced physical pleasure during sex, and clients would pay more to have condomless sex. Therefore, to maximise *monetary profit* (Bourdieu, 1986, p. 47) that was helping them to meet their personal and family needs, HYP engaged in condomless sex with clients. Thus, social obligations in intimate relationships, financial considerations, and power imbalances between HYP and clients produced a context of competing risks (Persson, 2013, p. 209) less conducive towards consistent condom use.

Nevertheless, HYP's cultural health capital (Shim, 2010) helped them to recognise that they were at risk of HIV/STIs. Here, peers helped HYP to acquire local knowledge of sexual safety, as they advised HYP to use methods like oral sex, masturbation, post-sex anal douching, and the use of specific sexual positions to protect against HIV/STIs. These methods were not always useful, and some of them might have inadvertently increased their risk of HIV infection.

References

Abid, M. J., Kumar, R., Khan, R., Ali, S., Chandra, P., Rani, R., & Khan, N. A. (2016). Assessment of Leucorrhea disease in female students. *Journal of Scientific and Innovative Research, 5*(4), 116–118.

Allahqoli, L., Fallahi, A., Rahmani, A., & Higgs, P. (2018). The prevalence of human immunodeficiency virus infection and the perceptions of sexually transmitted infections among homeless women. *Nursing & Midwifery Studies, 7*(4), 186–191.

Barker, J. D. (2016). A habitus of instability: Youth homelessness and instability. *Journal of Youth Studies, 19*(5), 665–683.

Bourdieu, P. (1984 [1979]). *Distinction: A social critique of the judgment of taste.* Harvard University Press.

Bourdieu, P. (1986). The forms of capital. In J. G. Richardson (Ed.), *Handbook of theory and research for the sociology* (pp. 241–258). Greenwood.

Buriro, A. A., & Endut, N. (2016). *Matchmaking and traditionally arranged marriages and domestic violence in Rural Sindh, Pakistan.* Paper presented at the 3rd Kanita postgraduate international conference on Gender Studies, Penang.

Busza, J. R., Balakireva, O. M., Teltschik, A., Bondar, T. V., Sereda, Y. V., Meynell, C., & Sakovych, O. (2011). Street-based adolescents at high risk of HIV in Ukraine. *Journal of Epidemiology and Community Health, 65*(12), 1166–1170.

Carballo-Dieguez, A., Bauermeister, J. A., Ventuneac, A., Dolezal, C., Balan, I., & Rehman, R. H. (2008). The use of rectal douches among HIV-uninfected and infected men who have unprotected receptive anal intercourse: Implications for rectal microbicides. *AIDS and Behavior, 12*(6), 860–866.

Dunn, J., Zhang, Q., Weeks, M. R., Li, J., Liao, S., & Li, F. (2017). Indigenous hiv prevention beliefs and practices among low-earning Chinese sex workers as context for introducing female condoms and other novel prevention options. *Qualitative Health Research, 27*(9), 1302–1315.

Gillmore, M. R., Archibald, M. E., Morrison, D. M., Wilsdon, A., Wells, E. A., Hoppe, M. J., ... Murowchick, E. (2002). Teen sexual behavior: Applicability of the theory of reasoned action. *Journal of Marriage and the Family, 64*(4), 885–897.

Green, A. I. (2008). The social organization of desire: The sexual fields approach. *Sociological Theory, 26*(1), 25.

Gross, G., & Tyring, S. K. (2011). *Sexually transmitted infections and sexually transmitted diseases.* Springer.

Hamid, S., Johansson, E., & Rubenson, B. (2011). Good parents' strive to raise 'innocent daughters. *Culture, Health & Sexuality, 13*(7), 841–851.

Jin, F., Jansson, J., Law, M., Prestage, G., Zaboltska, I., Imrie, J. C., ... Wilson, D. P. (2010). Per-contact probability of HIV transmission in homosexual men in Sydney in the era of HAART. *AIDS, 24*(6), 907–913.

Khan, M. S. (2011). *Poverty of opportunity for women selling sex in Lahore, Pakistan: Knowledge, experiences & magnitude of HIV & STIs.*

MacPhail, C., & Campbell, C. (2001). 'I think condoms are good but, aai, I hate those things':: Condom use among adolescents and young people in a Southern African township. *Social Science & Medicine, 52*(11), 1613–1627.

Millett, G. A., Peterson, J. L., Wolitski, R. J., & Stall, R. (2006). Greater risk for hiv infection of black men who have sex with men: A critical literature review. *American Journal of Public Health, 96*, 1007–1019.

Millett, G. A., Flores, S. A., Peterson, J. L., & Bakeman, R. (2007). Explaining disparities in HIV infection among black and white men who have sex with men: A meta-analysis of HIV risk behaviors. *AIDS, 21*, 2083–2091.

Noor, M. N., Holt, M., Qureshi, A., de Wit, J., & Bryant, J. (2020). Sexual risk-taking among homeless young people in Pakistan. *Health & Social Care in the Community, 00*, 1–9. https://doi.org/10.1111/hsc.13220

Persson, A. (2013). Notes on the concepts of 'serodiscordance' and 'risk' in couples with mixed HIV status. *Global Public Health, 8*(2), 209–220. https://doi.org/10.1080/1744169 2.2012.729219

Putnam, R. D. (1993). The prosperous community. *The American Prospect, 4*(*13*), 35–42.

Sherman, S. S., Plitt, S., ul Hassan, S., Cheng, Y., & Zafar, T. (2005). Drug use, street survival, and risk behaviors among street children in Lahore Pakistan. *Journal of Urban Health, 82*(Suppl 4), iv113–iv124.

Shim, J. K. (2010). Cultural health capital: A theoretical approach to understanding health care interactions and the dynamics of unequal treatment. *Journal of Health and Social Behavior, 51*(1), 1–15.

Tadele, G. (2010). "Boundaries of Sexual Safety": Men who have sex with men (MSM) and HIV/AIDS in Addis Ababa. *Journal of HIV/AIDS & Social Services, 9*(3), 261–280.

Toor, S. (2007). Moral regulation in a postcolonial nation-state. *Interventions, 9*(2), 255–275.

Van De Ven, P., Kippax, S., Crawford, J., Rawstorne, P., Prestage, G., Grulich, A., & Murphy, D. (2002). In a minority of gay men, sexual risk practice indicates strategic positioning for perceived risk reduction rather than unbridled sex. *AIDS Care, 14*(4), 471–480.

Vittinghoff, E., Douglas, J., Judson, F., McKirnan, D., MacQueen, K., & Buchbinder, S. P. (1999). Per-contact risk of human immunodeficiency virus transmission between male sexual partners. *American Journal of Epidemiology, 150*(3), 306–311.

Wacquant, L. J. (1998). Negative social capital: State breakdown and social destitution in America's urban core. *Netherlands Journal of Housing the Built Environment, 13*(1), 25.

Wang, B., Li, X., Stanton, B., Yang, H., Fang, X., Zhao, R., ... Liang, S. (2005). Vaginal douching, condom use, and sexually transmitted infections among Chinese female sex workers. *Sexually Transmitted Diseases, 32*(11), 696–702.

Warr, D. J. (2005). Social networks in a 'discredited' neighbourhood. *Journal of Sociology, 41*(3), 285–308.

Warwick, I., Aggleton, P., & Homans, H. (1988). Constructing commonsense—young people's beliefs about AIDS. *Sociology of Health & Illness, 10*(3), 213–233.

Zhao, J., Song, F., Ren, S., Wang, Y., Wang, L., Liu, W., ... Hu, T. (2012). Predictors of condom use behaviors based on the Health Belief Model (HBM) among female sex workers: A cross-sectional study in Hubei Province, China. *PLoS One, 7*(11), e49542.

Chapter 9
Key Messages and Implications for Health Promotion

This book contributes to the field of social research in health by providing new insights into the lived experiences of homeless young people (HYP) in Pakistan. Broadly speaking, using the theory of capital and social practice has helped to identify and explain social processes shaping HYP's pathways to homelessness, their journey on the streets, trajectories into sex work, and sexual choices, decisions, and practices, which may increase their risk of HIV and other sexually transmitted infections (STIs).

This final chapter is composed of four main sections. The first section highlights the key contributions of the study by synthesising the main findings and connecting them with existing literature on homelessness, sexual practice, and HIV. The second section discusses the limitations of this relatively small-scale study with some recommendations for researchers who may conduct future research into homelessness in Pakistan. The third section outlines the study's implications for policy and practice. Drawing on the *five action areas* of the Ottawa Charter for Health Promotion, it invites government and civil society organisations to take coordinated actions to address homelessness and HIV in Pakistan (WHO, 1986). The fourth section discusses implications for future research, which I propose should include further efforts to estimate the magnitude of homelessness and HIV prevalence among the homeless population in Pakistan and explore the relationship between heteronormativity, patriarchy, and homelessness. The chapter ends with a reminder that appropriate actions by the government and community-based organisations (CBOs) can help HYP in their efforts to contribute to the socio-economic development of Pakistan.

M. N. Noor, *Homeless Youth of Pakistan*, SpringerBriefs in Public Health,
https://doi.org/10.1007/978-3-030-79305-0_9

Key Contributions

This study is the most recent detailed social research that has examined the lived experiences of HYP in Pakistan. Generally, studies from Pakistan assume what Persson (2013, p. 212) calls a *linear relationship* between HIV/STI knowledge and HYP's sexual behaviour. The use of the theory of capital and social practice helps us to move beyond this narrow understanding that simply having biomedical knowledge can lead to safer sex practices (Bourdieu, 1984 [1979], 1986). Indeed, the theory enables us to identify how forms of capital produce conditions in which leaving the family home, living on the streets, practising sex work, and engaging in sexual risk-taking can become inevitable.

Using the concept of capital enabled me to analyse that a combination of structural and interpersonal forces produce unique conditions in which HYP take informed decisions. Many HYP were aware that they experienced a deficiency of financial capital – they left family homes with intentions to engage in paid work in an urban setting. Similarly, HYP, including cisgender women, transgender women, and gay men, who experienced violence, were aware that they lacked social capital within family settings – they chose to leave homes to secure social capital through which they could be protected. This indicates that HYP knew that they experienced significant social structural constraints, and this shaped their decision to prioritise things that they consider important: income generation, being openly transgender or gay (at least within peer groups), and avoiding violence.

Once on the streets, HYP looked for other options of support to accumulate needed social and financial capital. Contrary to the assumption that HYP *lack* social skills to navigate their lives, HYP's accounts of street life point to the agency they exercised in dealing with the significant social structural constraints they faced (Bahr & Caplow, 1968). The way HYP formed what I call the street field and how they operated within this terrain provides another evidence of their agency. The street field was organised around rules of inclusion and exclusion and the norms of trust and reciprocity, and this mechanism maintained the existence of the street field and the resources connected to it.

Another contribution of this study is its exposition of the benefits HYP derived from their relationship with intimate partners. Many HYP talked about how they had experienced emotional distress due to disrupted family life, experiences of discrimination, and ongoing social and financial insecurity. For them, intimate partners were the most valued source of respect, affection, and social support in an otherwise highly marginalised life. These findings support the view that intimate partnerships can help HYP to become accepted, recognised, and appreciated in an otherwise stigmatising and discriminatory environment (Blais et al., 2012; Kruks, 1991; Watson, 2011).

Noting that most of the HYP had concurrent sexual partnerships, the study explored the extent to which HYP practised safer sex. Contrary to past research that links insufficient STI-related knowledge with risky sexual behaviour, the study shows that most of the HYP often practised sex without condoms, although they knew about the risk of HIV/STIs (Allahqoli et al., 2018; Busza et al., 2011; Embleton et al., 2016). The findings indicate that HYP can supersede the risk of HIV/STIs in light of other pressing or more immediate considerations. For example, in intimate relationships, the risks of HIV/STIs were often secondary to concerns like physical protection and social and emotional security, which otherwise would be difficult to attain in a highly marginalised life. Moreover, due to the social and financial insecurity of HYP, avoiding violence from intoxicated clients and maximising their incomes took primacy over sexual health risks in sex work. This analysis supports the view that in contexts where competing risks are negotiated, HIV prevention can become a secondary concern (Persson, 2013; Prieur, 1990; Tadele, 2010).

Since HYP knew that they were at risk of HIV/STIs due to inconsistent condom use, they attempted to protect themselves with alternative strategies. Drawing on advice from peers, they used the withdrawal method and specific sexual positions and practised oral sex and post-sex douching, believing that these strategies would protect them from HIV. Unfortunately, these strategies were not always useful and might inadvertently increase their risk of HIV/STIs (Edward & Crane, 1998; Hawkins, 2001; Varghese et al., 2001).

Some Methodological Reflections

It would be appropriate to reflect on how the sensitive nature of the study topic and my position, being a relative outsider, may have influenced recruitment, interviewing, and the information obtained from HYP. Semi-structured interviews contained rich accounts of how HYP became homeless, what they did to navigate their social lives on the streets, with whom and why they practised sex, how the sexual practice helped them to secure various resources, and what contributed to their sexual risk-taking. However, it is possible that other aspects of their sexuality and sexual practices may not be known, given the sociocultural context in which the study was conducted. A small number of eligible HYP, including some lesbians (a sexually diverse population group that is missing in this study), refused to take part in the study, as they were not comfortable to provide information regarding their sexual experiences to someone who was an outsider (and a man). A study that could recruit peers as researchers could unearth more details regarding the interrelationship between sexuality, homelessness, and sexual practice. Also, many HYP in this study had a good knowledge of sexual health risks and condom use, perhaps because they were recruited through CBOs that were already working with them. HYP who are not connected with CBOs may not have much awareness of HIV/STIs, as documented by other survey-based studies from Pakistan (Ali et al., 2004; Emmanuel et al., 2005; Sherman et al., 2005). A multi-sited study with a large sample size can provide more insights into HYP's knowledge regarding HIV and sexual practices.

Implications for Policy and Practice

A range of structural- and interpersonal-level forces combinedly shaped HYP's pathways to homelessness, their street activities, and risky sexual behaviour. The best approaches to addressing complex, socially-produced health problems can be guided by the five action areas outlined in the Ottawa Charter for Health Promotion, including building healthy public policy, creating a supportive environment, strengthening community action, developing personal skills, and reorienting health services towards primary health care (WHO, 1986).

Building Healthy Public Policy

Building a healthy public policy means that policymakers need to promote legislation, fiscal measures, and organisational change to improve the lives of individuals (WHO, 1986). The results demonstrate a clear link between homelessness and risky sexual behaviour; it is important to consider why young people become homeless in the first place. Specifically, the relationship between poverty and homelessness indicates the need for actions taken to reduce poverty in Pakistan. Although various microfinance and charity programs aimed to reduce poverty in Pakistan, they are less effective largely because of inadequate investment and gaps in implementation (Ashraf, 2017). Poverty reduction is not an easy task, but a reconsideration of policies that underpin the existing microfinance programs may help to achieve better outcomes. In particular, adopting principles of a more successful microfinance program, like the Grameen Bank in Bangladesh, may help Pakistan to achieve better results in poverty reduction (Yunus, 2004).

Most of the HYP could not secure jobs in the formal market because they had limited education, and this suggests that actions are required to improve access to quality education. While Pakistan is constitutionally committed to providing free education up to Grade 10, poor parents often expect children to work to provide them with some financial support, which can lead to their discontinuation of education (Hazarika & Bedi, 2003; National Education Policy Framework, 2018). A government-supported cash transfer program – Waseela-e-Taleem (WeT) – has been encouraging poor parents to ensure their children's attendance 70% of the time at public schools to receive PKR 250 (about AUD$ 2.5)/month. The program has only been partially successful, as one million children of eligible households remained out of school and children who attended the schools also engaged in work to increase their families' incomes (Cheema et al., 2016). Perhaps aligning the WeT program's policies with more successful cash transfer programs in other developing countries may help to achieve better outcomes. Reviewing how OPORTUNIDADES and the Swa Koteka-HPTN have achieved better educational outcomes in Colombia and South Africa may help to revise the policies of the WeT program in Pakistan (Barrera-Osorio et al., 2011; MacPhail et al., 2018). For instance, the authorities of the WeT program could consider increasing the amount of cash transfer to students to allow them to focus on education. While limited economic resources in Pakistan can pose a challenge for the government to increase the cash transfer amount in the WeT program, additional support from international bodies like the World Bank (which is already supporting the WeT program) could help to achieve this goal.

Creating a Supportive Environment

Creating environments that can enable individuals to take control of the social determinants of their health can promote good health. As can be seen from the findings, HYP practised sex in environments that were not conducive to using condoms consistently. For instance, HYP often engage in condomless sex because they believed that it could affect their relationship with intimate partners. Sexual health-promoting organisations might encourage HYP to bring their intimate partners to attend sexual health education sessions. This could help intimate partners to consider achieving good health as a mutual responsibility, which could increase their condom use.

Since clients may not want to reveal their identity by meeting staff from health promotion organisations, a useful way to educate them could be the use of information, education, and communication (IEC) material. As most HYP practised sex at rooms they temporarily rented, it might be useful to encourage them to display posters on walls and make leaflets available that contain information about HIV transmission, prevention, testing, and treatment to clients.

To deal with violent clients who compel HYP to have condomless sex, it is important to develop a support mechanism that can empower them. HYP revealed how the police sometimes received protection money to allow them to practise sex work. This shows that despite its illegality, sex work is practised and recognised as an 'open secret' in Pakistan (Emmanuel et al., 2013, p. ii29). Therefore, making political, legal, and institutional authorities aware of the relationship between homelessness, sex work, and HIV could help the police support HYP in dealing with violent clients, although it is a complex challenge. There is evidence that despite the illegality of sex work, Pakistan has recognised, to some extent, the health needs of male, female, and transgender sex workers and provided them sexual health education and medical care to decrease their risk of HIV (Rajabali et al., 2008).

Strengthening Community Actions

At the heart of community empowerment is the recognition of individuals' fundamental rights and enabling their access to adequate information, resources, and social support (WHO, 1986). The present study identifies how the denial of HYP's fundamental rights to receive education, enter the formal job market, and be accepted as a person with a diverse sexual or gender identity has systematically put them at risk of HIV. Putting homelessness and HIV on the agenda of civil society organisations can help to address the needs of young people. There is evidence that civil society organisations have promoted women and transgender rights by sensitising political and legal authorities in Pakistan, which also resulted in the issuance of transgender passports and promoting formal education among them (Haider, 2017; Khan, 2014; The Express Tribune, 2019; Transgender Persons (Protection of Rights) act, 2018). Although these actions indicate a political commitment towards the acceptance and empowerment of women and the transgender community, they still experience discrimination and violence from society (Alizai et al., 2017). Here, it may be useful for organisations like the Human Rights Commission of Pakistan (HRCP) and the Aurat (woman) Foundation to promote tolerance and gender equality through media campaigns.

Developing Personal Skills

The Ottawa Charter suggests that health promotion should also enhance individuals' skills to enable them to cope with health-related and other social problems they may face in their lives (WHO, 1986). The fact that HYP displayed agency within significant constraints indicates their resourcefulness. Providing HYP with vocational education could help them to utilise their abilities in a positive direction and open avenues to the formal job market. CBOs might also need to consider linking HYP with vocational institutes that operate in almost all districts of Pakistan and offer short courses related to beautification, dress designing and making, information technology, office management, and other technical and mechanical skills (UNESCO, 2015). Conditional cash transfers could encourage young people to attend the institutes, which could help them secure socially accepted jobs, further contributing to their social inclusiveness.

Reorienting Health Services

Health services should also participate in health promotion rather than merely treating diseases (WHO, 1986). In the present study, HYP largely received sexual health education and medical care from a few CBOs with limited resources and infrastructure, rather than from the government health services. Pakistan is one of the initial signatories of the WHO Alma-Ata Declaration and, hence, is committed to promoting health among its citizens (Ronis & Nishtar, 2007). However, child immunisation, family planning, and maternal health promotion programs have largely been the focus of health promotion in the country. Since 1994, the Lady Health Worker Program (LHWP) has contributed to improved contraceptive use and maternal and child health in Pakistan (Zhu et al., 2014). Nevertheless, few efforts have been made to promote sexual health in the country (Talpur & Khowaja, 2012). The government might also consider deploying male health workers and connect them and the lady health workers with the National AIDS Control Program to prevent HIV among HYP and their counterparts.

Implications for Future Research

Since it is not possible to adequately address homelessness unless the magnitude of this problem is known, the next population census of Pakistan could estimate the number of HYP in the country. Furthermore, researchers should conduct surveys to estimate the prevalence of homelessness in major urban centres of Pakistan. Also, estimating the number of those who are precariously housed can help policymakers to know the size of the population at risk of homelessness and devise actions to address this issue. A few HYP reportedly contracted genital rashes, herpes, and gonorrhoea, and one homeless young man reported an HIV diagnosis. There is also evidence of an increased prevalence of HIV among HYP in other countries (Braitstein et al., 2018; Skyers et al., 2018). The next integrated behavioural and biological surveillance in Pakistan could include HYP as a key population, which would have implications for the National AIDS Control Program. The biological surveillance of HYP has been useful to identify the growing number of HIV cases in other countries (Towe et al., 2019).

This is also the most recent study based on cross-sectional research designed to highlight the relationship between heteronormativity, homelessness, and sexual behaviour in the context of Pakistan. Conducting longitudinal research into how heteronormativity can give various shapes to the lives of young people with diverse sexual and gender identities can provide rich information, which can be useful in sensitising political and legal authorities to take actions towards their social inclusiveness.

Conclusion

The study's exposition of risky sexual practices of HYP is a reminder that HIV should not be reduced to the context of brothel-based sex work. It is necessary to understand the social conditions that shape individuals' sexual practices that put them at increased risk for HIV. Therefore, the conventional approach of promoting health through raising awareness regarding sexual health risks may continue to bring less than promising outcomes unless we focus on how macro-structures operate and increase the chances of risky sex. The fact that young people in the present study displayed agency within significant social structural constraints reflects their resilience and efforts to improve their social and financial status. Together, policymakers, academics, and civil society organisations can help young people utilise their abilities in productive ways to further contribute to the socio-economic development of Pakistan, a country where young people make up over half of the population.

What, then, have I learned by conducting this social scientific research? I think this research has significantly contributed to my understanding of the relationships between social conditions, marginalisation, sexual practice, and HIV/STIs. Increasing populations' biomedical knowledge regarding HIV/STIs is important, as it supports their evaluation of risk. However, the social scientific approach taken in this study enabled me to move beyond the narrow understanding that biomedical knowledge alone can lead to safer sex practices. Indeed, I am now more cognisant of how broader social structures operate and often affect population groups' vulnerability to poverty, abuse, stigma, and social exclusion, all of which are directly or indirectly linked with sexual risk-taking. In Pakistan, as well as in other country contexts, people who inject drugs, sex workers, men who have sex with men, and, sometimes, HYP are categorised as being at high risk of HIV. However, the social conditions that place them at risk of HIV are often ignored when it comes to health promotion, as are their unique intersecting identities, which can affect their health outcomes in many ways. Having completed this research, I think that the next thing I must do is to contribute to HIV/STI prevention efforts in Pakistan. I can do this by highlighting, through research, writing, advocacy, and activism, how social structural issues like poverty, gender inequality, and domestic violence continue to complicate HIV prevention efforts.

References

Ali, M., Shahab, S., Ushijima, S., & de Muynck, A. (2004). Street children in Pakistan: A situational analysis of social conditions and nutritional status. *Social Science & Medicine, 59*, 1707–1717.

Alizai, A., Doneys, P., & Doane, D. L. (2017). Impact of gender binarism on Hijras' life course and their access to fundamental human rights in Pakistan. *Journal of Homosexuality, 64*(9), 1214–1240.

Allahqoli, L., Fallahi, A., Rahmani, A., & Higgs, P. (2018). The prevalence of human immunodeficiency virus infection and the perceptions of sexually transmitted infections among homeless women. *Nursing & Midwifery Studies, 7*(4), 186–191.

Ashraf, M. A. (2017). Poverty and its alleviation: The case of Pakistan. In G. L. Staicu (Ed.), *Poverty, inequality and policy.*

Bahr, H. M., & Caplow, T. (1968). Homelessness, affiliation, and occupational mobility. *Social Forces, 47*(1), 28–33.

Barrera-Osorio, F., Bertrand, M., Linden, L. L., & Perez-Calle, F. (2011). Improving the design of conditional transfer programs: Evidence from a randomized education experiment in Colombia. *American Economic Journal: Applied Economics, 3*(2), 167–195.

Blais, M., Côté, P. B., Manseau, H., Martel, M., & Provencher, M. A. (2012). Love without a home: a portrait of romantic and couple relationships among street-involved young adults in Montreal. *Journal of Youth Studies, 15*(4), 403–420.

Bourdieu, P. (1984 [1979]). *Distinction: A social critique of the judgment of taste.* Cambridge: Harvard University Press.

Bourdieu, P. (1986). The forms of capital. In J. G. Richardson (Ed.), *Handbook of theory and research for the sociology* (pp. 241–258). Greenwood.

Braitstein, P., Ayuku, D., DeLong, A., Makori, D., Sang, E., Tarus, E., … Wachira, J. (2018). HIV prevalence in young people and children living on the streets, Kenya. *Bulletin of the World Health Organization, 97,* 33–41.

Busza, J. R., Balakireva, O. M., Teltschik, A., Bondar, T. V., Sereda, Y. V., Meynell, C., & Sakovych, O. (2011). Street-based adolescents at high risk of HIV in Ukraine. *Journal of Epidemiology and Community Health, 65*(12), 1166–1170.

Cheema, I., Asia, M. G., Hunt, S., Javeed, S., Lone, T., & O'Leary, S. (2016). *Benazir income support programme evaluation of the Waseela-e-Taleem conditional cash transfer.* Retrieved from Islamabad:

Edward, S., & Crane, C. (1998). Oral sex and the transmission if viral STIs. *Sexually Transmitted Infections, 74*(1), 6–10.

Embleton, L., Wachira, J., Kamanda, A., Naanyu, V., Ayuku, D., & Braitstein, P. (2016). Eating sweets without the wrapper: perceptions of HIV and sexually transmitted infections among street youth in western Kenya. *Culture, Health & Sexuality, 18*(3), 337–348.

Emmanuel, F., Iqbal, F., & Khan , N. (2005). *Street children in Pakistan: a group at risk of HIV/ AIDS.* Retrieved from Pakistan:

Emmanuel, F., Thompson, L. H., Athar, U., Salim, S., Sonia, A., Akhtar, N., & Blanchard, J. F. (2013). The organisation, operational dynamics and structure of female sex work in Pakistan. *Sexually Transmitted Infections, 89,* ii29–ii33.

Haider, Z. (2017). Pakistan issues landmark transgender passport; fight for rights goes on.

Hawkins, D. A. (2001). Oral sex and HIV transmission. *Sexually Transmitted Infections, 77*(5), 307–308.

Hazarika, G., & Bedi, A. (2003). Schooling costs and child work in rural Pakistan. *The Journal of Development Studies, 39*(5), 29–64.

Khan, F. A. (2014). Khwaja Sira: Culture, identity politics, and "transgender" activism in Pakistan. .

Kruks, G. (1991). Gay and lesbian homeless/street youth: special issues and concern. *Journal of Adolescent Health, 12*(7), 515–518.

MacPhail, C., Khoza, N., Selin, A., Julien, A., Twine, R., Wagner, R. G., … Pettifor, A. (2018). Cash transfer for HIV prevention: What do young women spend it on? Mixed methods findings from HPTN 068. *BMC Public Health, 18*(1), 10.

National Education Policy Framework. (2018). *National education policy framework.* Retrieved from http://aserpakistan.org/document/2018/National_Eductaion_Policy_Framework_2018_ Final.pdf

Persson, A. (2013). Notes on the concepts of 'serodiscordance' and 'risk' in couples with mixed HIV status. *Global Public Health, 8*(2), 209–220. https://doi.org/10.1080/1744169 2.2012.729219

Prieur, A. (1990). Norwegian gay men: Reasons for continued practice of unsafe sex. *AIDS Education and Prevention, 2*(2), 109–115.

Rajabali, A., Khan, S., Warraich, H. J., Khanani, M. R., & Ali, S. H. (2008). HIV and homosexuality in Pakistan. *Infectious Diseases, 8*(8), 511–515.

Ronis, K. A., & Nishtar, S. (2007). Community health promotion in Pakistan: A policy development perspective. *Promotion & Education, 14*(2), 98–99.

Sherman, S. S., Plitt, S., ul Hassan, S, Cheng, Y., & Zafar, T. (2005). Drug use, street survival, and risk behaviors among street children in Lahore Pakistan. *Journal of Urban Health, 82*(Suppl 4), iv113–iv124.

Skyers, N., Jarrett, S., McFarland, W., Cole, D., & Atkinson, U. (2018). HIV risk and gender in Jamaica's homeless population. *AIDS and Behavior, 22,* S65–S69.

Tadele, G. (2010). "Boundaries of Sexual Safety": Men who have sex with men (MSM) and HIV/ AIDS in Addis Ababa. *Journal of HIV/AIDS & Social Services, 9*(3), 261–280.

Talpur, A. A., & Khowaja, A. R. (2012). Awareness and attitude towards sex health education and sexual health services among youngsters in rural and urban settings of Sindh, Pakistan. *The Journal of the Pakistan Medical Association, 62*(7), 708–712.

The Express Tribune. (2019). *Pakistan's first public school for transgender persons opens doors in Lodhran.* Retrieved from https://tribune.com.pk/story/1917540/1-pakistans-first-public-school-transgender-persons-opens-doors-lodhran/

Towe, V. L., Wiewel, E. W., Zhong, Y., Linnemayr, S., Johnson, R., & Rojass, J. (2019). A randomized controlled trial of a rapid re-housing intervention for homeless persons living with HIV/AIDS: Impact on housing and HIV medical outcomes. *AIDS and Behavior, 23*, 2315.

Transgender Persons (Protection of Rights) act. (2018). Retrieved from http://www.na.gov.pk/uploads/documents/1526547582_234.pdf

UNESCO. (2015). *World TVET database Pakistan.* Retrieved from https://unevoc.unesco.org/wtdb/worldtvetdatabase_pak_en.pdf

Varghese, B., Maher, J. E., Peterman, T. A., Branson, B. M., & Steketee, W. (2001). Reducing the risk of sexual HIV transmission. quantifying the per-act risk for HIV on the basis of choice of partner, sex act, and condom use. *Sexually Transmitted Diseases, 29*(1), 38–43.

Watson, J. (2011). Understanding survival sex: young women, homelessness and intimate relationships. *Journal of Youth Studies, 14*(6), 639–655.

WHO (Producer). (1986). *The Ottawa charter for health promotion.* Retrieved from https://www.who.int/healthpromotion/conferences/previous/ottawa/en/index1.html

Yunus, M. (2004). Grameen bank, microcredit, and Millennium Development Goals. *Economic and Political Weekly, 39*(36), 4077–4080.

Zhu, N., Allen, E., Kearns, A., Caglia, J., & Atun, R. (2014). *Lady health workers in Pakistan, Improving access to health care for rural women and families.* Retrieved from

Index

Printed in the United States
by Baker & Taylor Publisher Services